# CHRISTMAS IN PU[RGATORY]

## A Photographic Essay on Mental Retardation

**BURTON BLATT**
Syracuse University
Centennial Professor and
Director, Division of Special
Education and Rehabilitation

**FRED KAPLAN**
Black Star Corporation

Foreword by

**SEYMOUR B. SARASON**
Professor of Psychology
Yale University

HUMAN POLICY PRESS / SYRACUSE, NEW YORK / 1974

Dedicated to
those who made this book possible

Library of Congress Catalog Card Number: 66-25682.

Printed in the United States of America.

Previously published by Allyn and Bacon, Inc., 1966

# FOREWORD

The contents, verbal and visual, of this book produced little surprise for me. Initially, it brought back memories of a number of visits I made to various institu- tions twenty-five years ago when I first began to work in the field of mental retar- dation. As the years went on, it became increasingly clear to me that the conditions I saw—and which are documented in this book—were not due to evil, incompetent or cruel people but rather to a concept of human potential and an attitude toward innovation which when applied to the mentally defective, result in a self-fulfilling prophecy. That is, if one thinks that defective children are almost beyond help, one acts toward them in ways which then confirm one's assumptions. This is similar to the situation several decades ago when, in many psychiatric hospitals, the diagnosis of schizophrenia contained the prognosis that the sick patients would never improve. That most of these patients did not improve did not reflect the validity of the diagnosis, but the dishearteningly effective way in which state hospitals unwittingly went about confirming their diagnosis. In contrasting one institution (The Seaside), which views the defective child in one way, with other institutions which hold to another viewpoint, the authors have incisively made the point that the basic problem is in the realm of concept of human behavior and its amenability to change under specified conditions.

I would not deny that increased appropriations will make for better physical care. But spending more money is easy compared to the problem of how one gets people to change their concepts and to view innovation and experimentation as necessities rather than as subversive suggestions or the terminal points of the meandering of the academic mind.

Dr. Blatt is an eminent educator, and the reader unfamiliar with his work can be assured that this book reflects the conscientious research of a well-informed man vitally concerned with human welfare in general, and specifically, the problems of mental retardation and institutions. He has been under great pressure from many quarters to reveal the names of the institutions visited, but for reasons made plain on the pages which follow, Dr. Blatt would not go back on promises made to those persons who permitted him to make this study. He wished, also, in not naming names, to avoid creating the impression that this problem is a local rather than a national one.

Seymour B. Sarason
Yale University

# PREFACE

The first edition of this book was published in August, 1966, and was distributed without charge under the auspices of a group of parents and friends of the mentally retarded. These thousand copies were sent to prominent legislators, commissioners of mental health, university professors, and leaders in the parent movement in mental retardation. The response to the first volume was overwhelming, leading to the present Allyn and Bacon edition.

The purpose of this book is to present our findings in the hope that they will inspire constructive action among those in responsible positions. For those not in positions to legislate or reform, we hope to strike a chord of awareness, to shatter the shell of complacency born of ignorance that surrounds the problem. From this element of society, we hope for support. The first section of this essay represents conditions existing in too many institutions for the retarded. The second section of the book is devoted to the heartening conditions we found at The Seaside. Our optimism for the betterment of state institutions is based on the evidence of the forward strides that have been made there. To us, The Seaside represents what can be done with funds, intelligent administration and an adequate, sensitive and well-trained staff.

We cannot permit ourselves thoughts of immediate radical reform as a result of our efforts. We can only hope for increased public interest. As Camus once wrote: "Perhaps we cannot stop the world from being one in which children are tortured, but we can reduce the number of children tortured."

*iii*

When a commercial publisher discontinues, as in this case, publication of a book it is because it is no longer profitable. This does not necessarily mean that people do not want to buy the book. It can mean that the escalating costs of printing and promotion—and, of course, the need to maintain certain profit levels—put the costs of the book out of the reach of most people, e.g., students. (Fairness requires that I acknowledge the fact that the previous publisher was the only one willing to take a chance with so "different" a book.) Some extraordinary good books have sunk into oblivion. It would have been immoral, or at least an adverse commentary on our societal values, if **Christmas In Purgatory** was allowed to be available only in libraries (those which have copies). For one thing, this is an historical document. It was extraordinarily "profitable" in terms of its international influence on thinking, values, practices, and planning (not, ironically, in Dr. Blatt's home state where huge building complexes for the retarded continue to be developed). It was a simple, easily grasped, compelling, upsetting visual document which stood as a reminder of what existed in our society, and as a criterion by which to judge any derivative of our propensity to segregate people who are or look "different." It is noteworthy that in the last book, **Souls in Extremis**, Dr. Blatt concludes that purgatory is inherent in our concept of institutions, and he recommends that we close them and build no more. Precisely because institutional purgatories exist today and will continue to exist for the foreseeable future, **Christmas In Purgatory** should continue to be available. We should be grateful that it will be.

Seymour B. Sarason
Yale University

# INTRODUCTION

> "They cover a dung hill with a piece of
> tapestry when a procession goes by."
>
> Miguel de Cervantes

There is a hell on earth, and in America there is a special inferno. We were visitors there during Christmas, 1965.

During the early fall of that year, United States Senator Robert Kennedy visited several of his state's institutions for the mentally retarded. His reactions to these visits were widely published in our news media. These disclosures shocked millions of Americans and infuriated scores of public office holders and professional persons responsible for the care and treatment of the mentally retarded.

A segment of the general public was numbed because it is difficult for the "uninvolved" people to believe that in our country, today, human beings are being treated less humanely, with less care, and under more deplorable conditions than animals. A number of the "involved" citizenry—i.e. those who legislate and budget for the institutions for the mentally retarded and those who administer them—were infuriated because the Senator reacted only to the worst of what he had seen, not to the worthwhile programs that he might have. Further, this latter group was severely critical of the Senator for taking "whirlwind" tours and, in the light of just a few hours of observation, damning entire institutions and philosophies.

During the time of these visits I was a participant in a research project at The Seaside, a State of Connecticut Regional Center for the mentally retarded. The superintendent of The Seaside, Fred Finn, and I spent a considerable amount of time discussing the debate between Senator Kennedy and his Governor, Nelson Rockefeller. We concluded the following. It does not require a scientific background or a great deal of observation to determine that one has entered the "land of the living dead." It does not require too imaginative a mind or too sensitive a proboscis to realize that one has stumbled into a dung hill, regardless of how it is camouflaged. It is quite irrelevant how well the rest of an institution's program is being fulfilled if one is concerned about that part of it which is terrifying. No amount of rationalization can mitigate that which, to many of us, is cruel and inhuman treatment.

It is true that a short visit to the back wards of an institution for the mentally retarded will not provide, even for the most astute observer, any clear notion of the antecedents of the problems observed, the complexities of dealing with them, or ways to correct them. We can believe that the Senator did not fully comprehend the subtleties, the tenuous relationships, the grossness of budgetary inequities, the long history of political machinations, the extraordinary difficulty in providing care for severely mentally retarded patients, the unavailability of highly trained professional leaders, and the near-impossibility in recruiting dedicated attendants and ward personnel. But, we know, as well as do thousands of others who have been associated with institutions for the mentally retarded, that what Senator Kennedy claimed to have seen he did see. In fact, we know personally of few institutions for the mentally retarded in the United States completely free of dirt and filth, odors, naked patients groveling in their own feces, children in locked cells, horribly crowded dormitories, and understaffed and wrongly staffed facilities.

After a good deal of thought, I decided to follow through on a seemingly bizarre venture. One of my close friends, Fred Kaplan, is a freelance photographer who has worked for many national publications. The following plan was presented to him. We were to arrange to meet with each of several key administrative persons in a variety of public institutions for the mentally retarded. If we gained an individual's cooperation, in spite of the obvious great risk he would be assuming with respect to his institutional status and possible job security, we would be taken on a "tour" of the back wards and those parts of the institution that he was <u>most</u> ashamed of. On the "tour" Fred Kaplan would take pictures of what we observed, utilizing a hidden camera attached to his belt. During the month of December, 1965, we visited—at our own expense—five state institutions for the mentally retarded in four eastern states. Through the efforts of courageous and humanitarian colleagues, including two superintendents who put their reputations and professional positions in jeopardy, we were able to visit the darkest corridors and vestibules that humanity provides for its journey to purgatory and, without being detected by ward personnel and professional staff, Fred Kaplan was able to take hundreds of photographs.

The latter point deserves some comment. Our photographs are not always the clearest and, probably, Fred Kaplan is not proud of the technical qualities of every one published in this book. On the other hand, it required a truly creative and skilled photographer to take these pictures, "from the hip" so to speak, unable to use special lighting, not permitted to focus or set shutter speeds, with a small camera concealed in multitudes of clothing and surrounded by innumerable "eyes" of patients as well as of staff. Although our pictures could not even begin to capture a total and overwhelming horror we saw, smelled, and felt, they represent a side of America that has rarely been shown to the general public and is little understood by most of us.

We do not believe it is necessary to disclose the names of the institutions we visited. First, we have a deep debt of gratitude to those who permitted us to photograph that which <u>they</u> are most ashamed of. To reveal the names of the places we visited is, assuredly, an invitation to invite their instant dismissal. However, we have a much more forceful reason for not admitting to where we have been. These pictures are a challenge to all institutions for the mentally retarded in the United States. We are firmly convinced that in many other institutions in America we could have taken the same pictures—some, we are sure, even more frightening.

Our "Christmas in Purgatory" brought us to the depths of despair. We now have a deep sorrow, one that will not abate until the American people are aware of—and do something about—the treatment of the severely mentally retarded in our state institutions. We have again been caused to realize that "Man's inhumanity to man makes countless thousands mourn."

It is fitting that this book—our purgatory in black and white—was written on the 700th anniversary of the birth of Dante.

B.B.

# "Abandon all hope..."

"Abandon all hope, ye who enter here."

Dante

This book is divided into two major sections. The first section covers our visits to four institutions for the mentally retarded, located in three eastern states. The second section describes a fifth institution in another state. The latter is our way of communicating our deep conviction that many of the severe conditions with which you are about to become involved are not necessary consequences of the fact of institutionalization of mentally retarded individuals. These problems are largely the result of inadequate budgets, inferior facilities, untrained personnel, and haphazard planning—in spite of some dedicated and skilled professional workers in each of the institutions we visited. For example, the average per capita daily cost for maintaining a retarded resident in each of the four institutions we are about to describe is less than $7.00 and, in one state school, less than $5.00. In contrast, The Seaside, a regional center for the retarded sponsored by the Connecticut Department of Health, spends $12.00 daily for the care and treatment of each resident.

As was mentioned in the foreword, we are not disclosing the names of either of the institutions or the states where they are located with the exception of—for obvious reasons—the contrast institution. As far as the contrast institution, The Seaside, is concerned, we will be speaking about that one Center. We make no claim that The Seaside is representative or not representative of the Connecticut program for the mentally retarded although the State of Connecticut is to be commended for this—at least one—affirmation of the dignity of all mankind.

We repeat something already said, needing emphasis. What was observed in the institutions presented in Part I reflects what we have seen in other state institutions for the mentally retarded in other parts of the country. We know of few state institutions that do not—to a degree—have problems similar to the ones discussed in this book. The Seaside is one of the rare examples where one may see every ward—without becoming revolted or depressed. To be sure, every institution we visited during our Christmas recess had many things of which to be proud and further, each is accomplishing good work in the care and treatment. However, with the exception of The Seaside, each had made miniscule progress, especially in those areas concerning the care of severely retarded ambulatory adults and moderately and severely retarded young children. It is in the hope of calling attention to the desperate needs of these institutions and thereby paving the way for upgrading all institutions for the mentally retarded in all dimensions of their responsibilities that this study was undertaken.

Several things strike the visitor to most institutions for the mentally retarded upon his arrival. Often there are fences. Sometimes with barbed wire. Frequently the buildings impress him with their massiveness and impenetrability. We have observed bars on windows and locks—many locks—on inside as well as outside doors.

As we entered the dormitories and other buildings, we were impressed with the contrast of the functional superiority of the new buildings and the gross neglect of the older buildings. We have observed gaping holes in ceilings of the main kitchen. In toilets, one sees urinals ripped out, sinks broken, and toilets backed up.

In every institution discussed in this section, we found incredible overcrowding. Beds are so arranged—side by side and head to head—that it is impossible, in some dormitories, to cross parts of the rooms without actually walking over beds. Often the beds are without pillows. We have seen mattresses so sagged by the weight of bodies that they were scraping the floor.

In summary, we were amazed by the overcrowdedness, by the disrepair of older buildings, by the excessive use of locks and heavy doors, and by the enormity of buildings and numbers of patients assigned to dormitories.

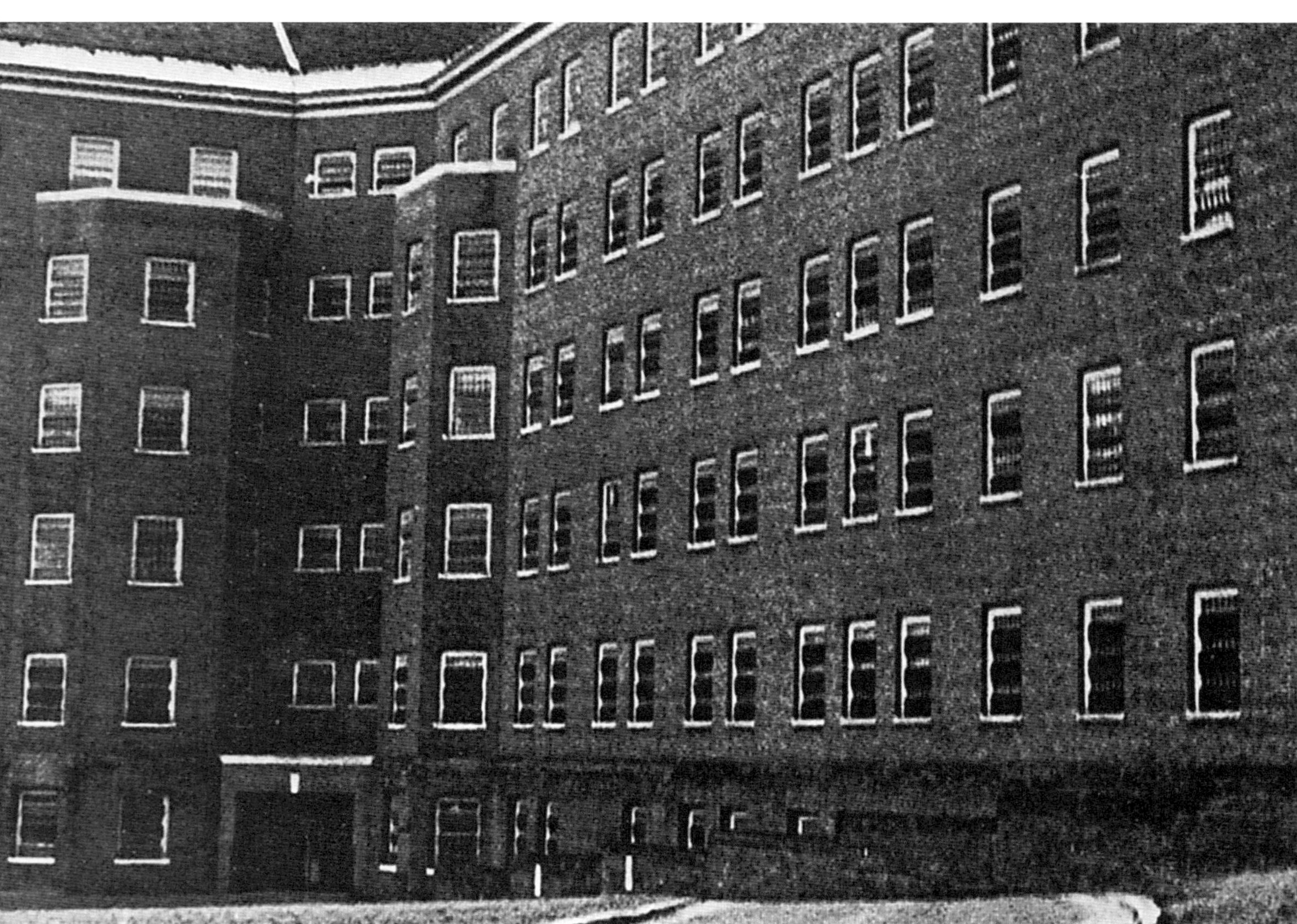

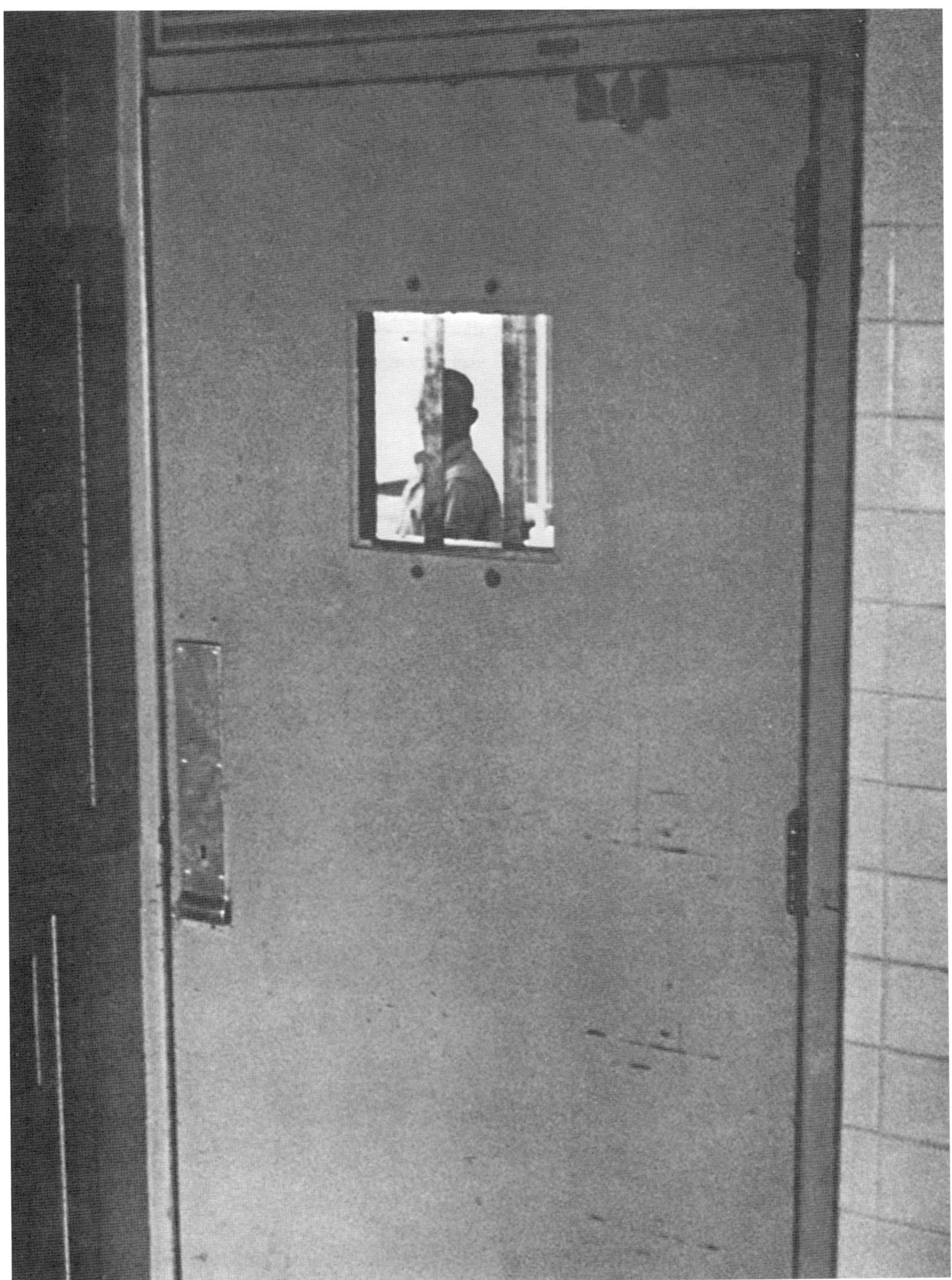

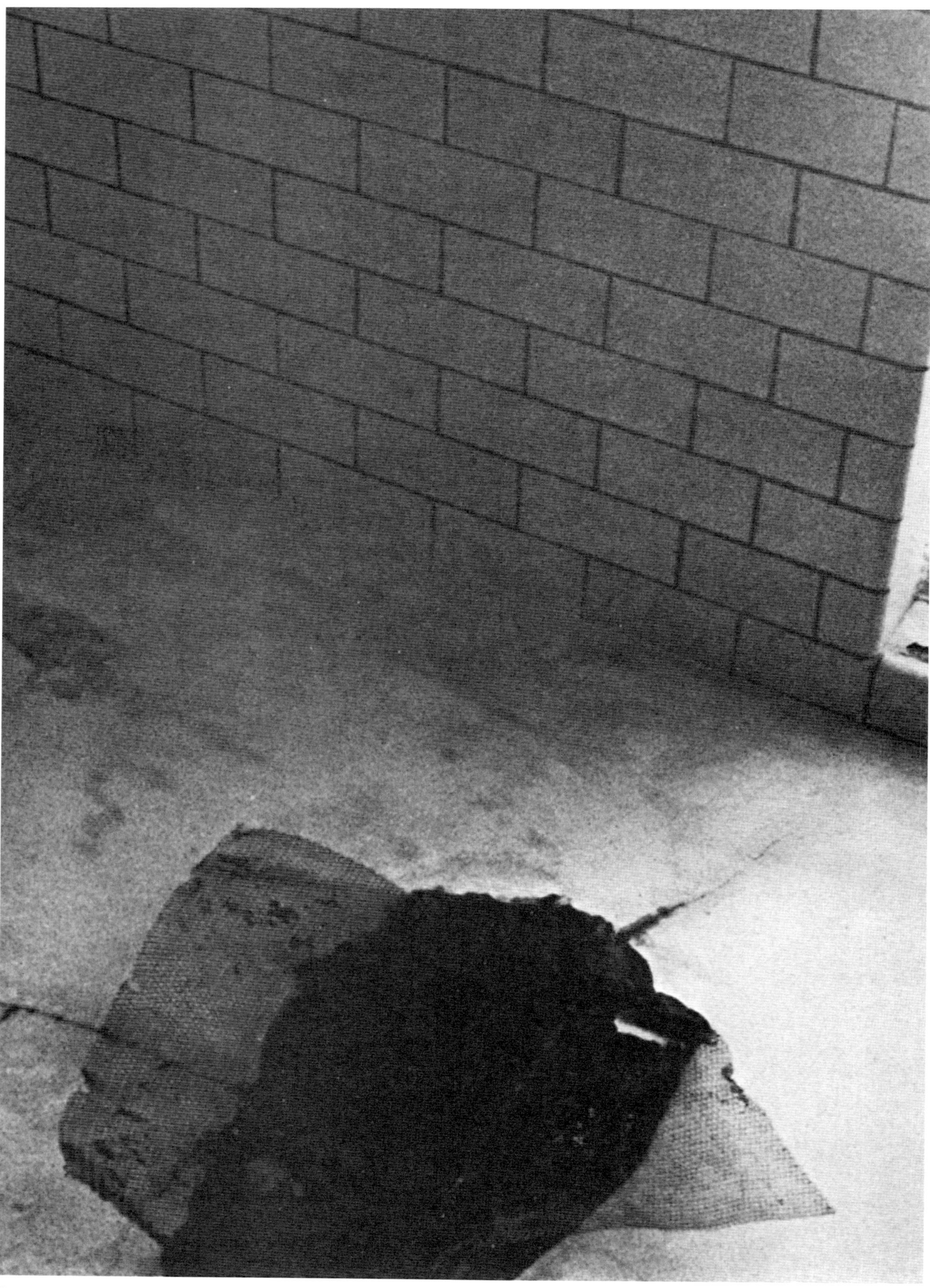

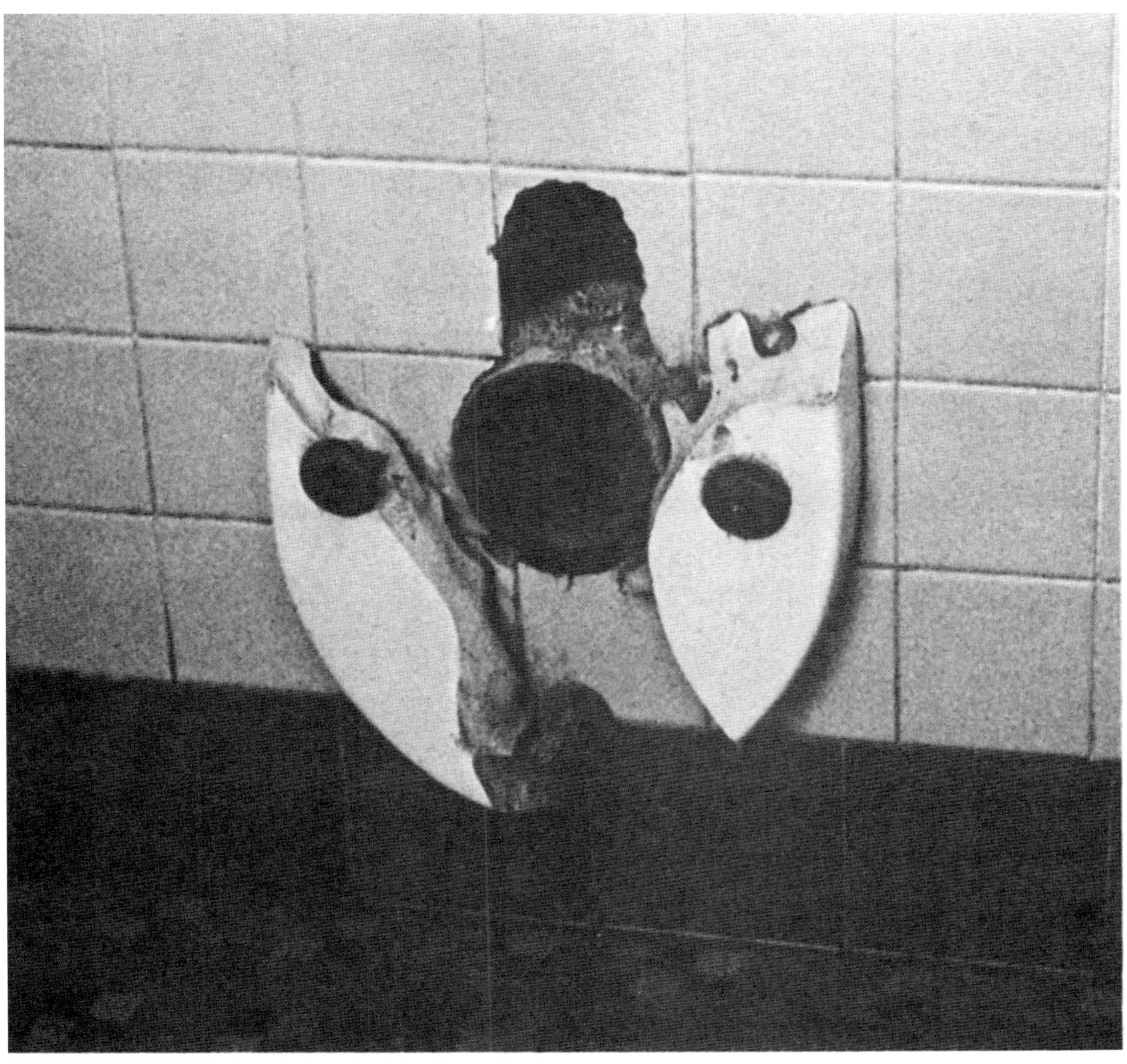

"There is a wide range among the States in the cost per day spent for the care of the mentally retarded. Six States spent less than $2.50 a day per patient, while only seven States spent over $5.50 per day. Nationally, the average is $4.55 per day, less than one-sixth of the amounts spent for general hospital care."

The President's Panel on
Mental Retardation

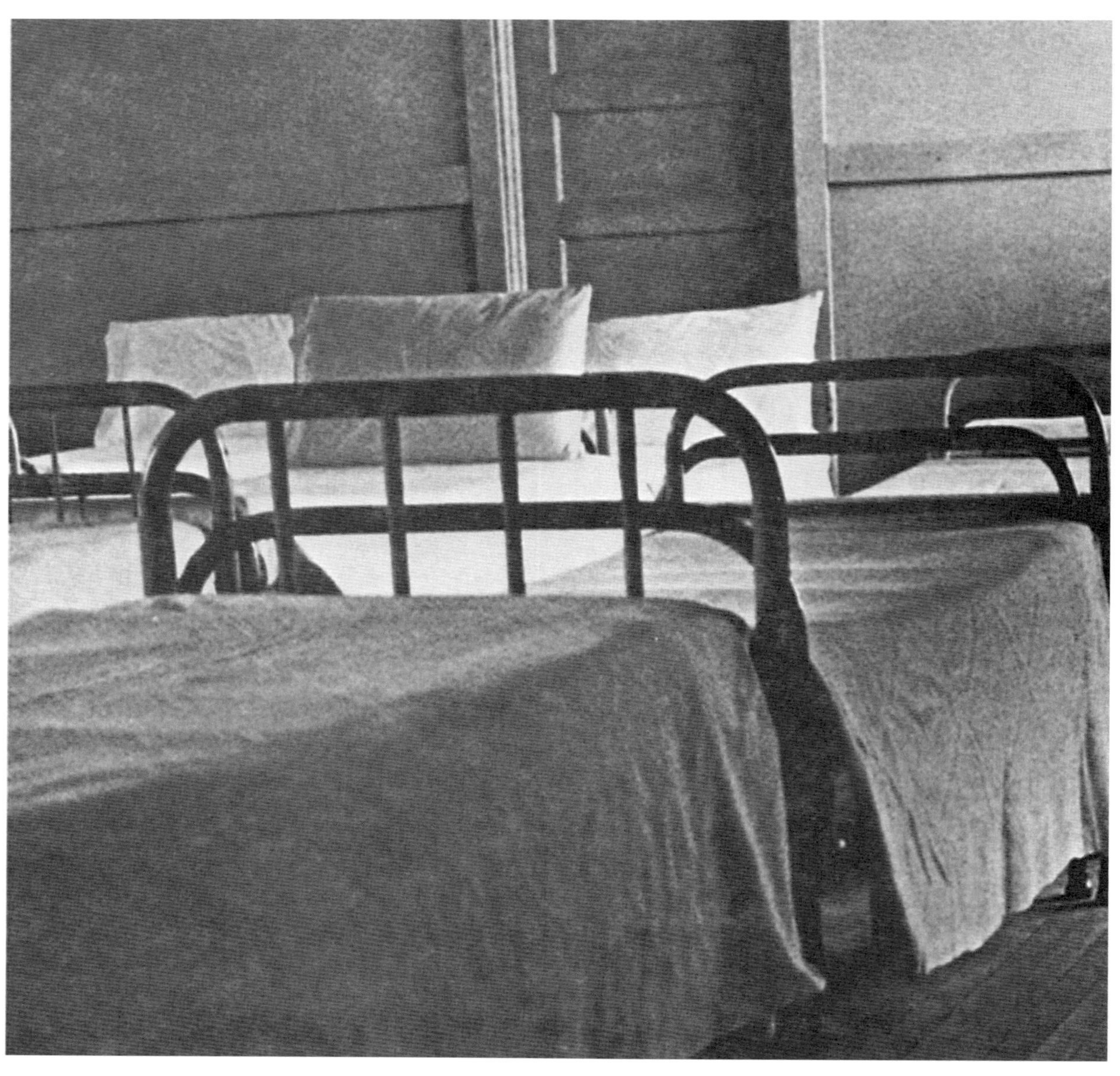

"The population of State residential facilities runs the gamut from a few hundred to more than 5,000; but on the average, each institution is caring for 350 patients over state capacity and has a waiting list of better than 300."

The President's Panel on
Mental Retardation

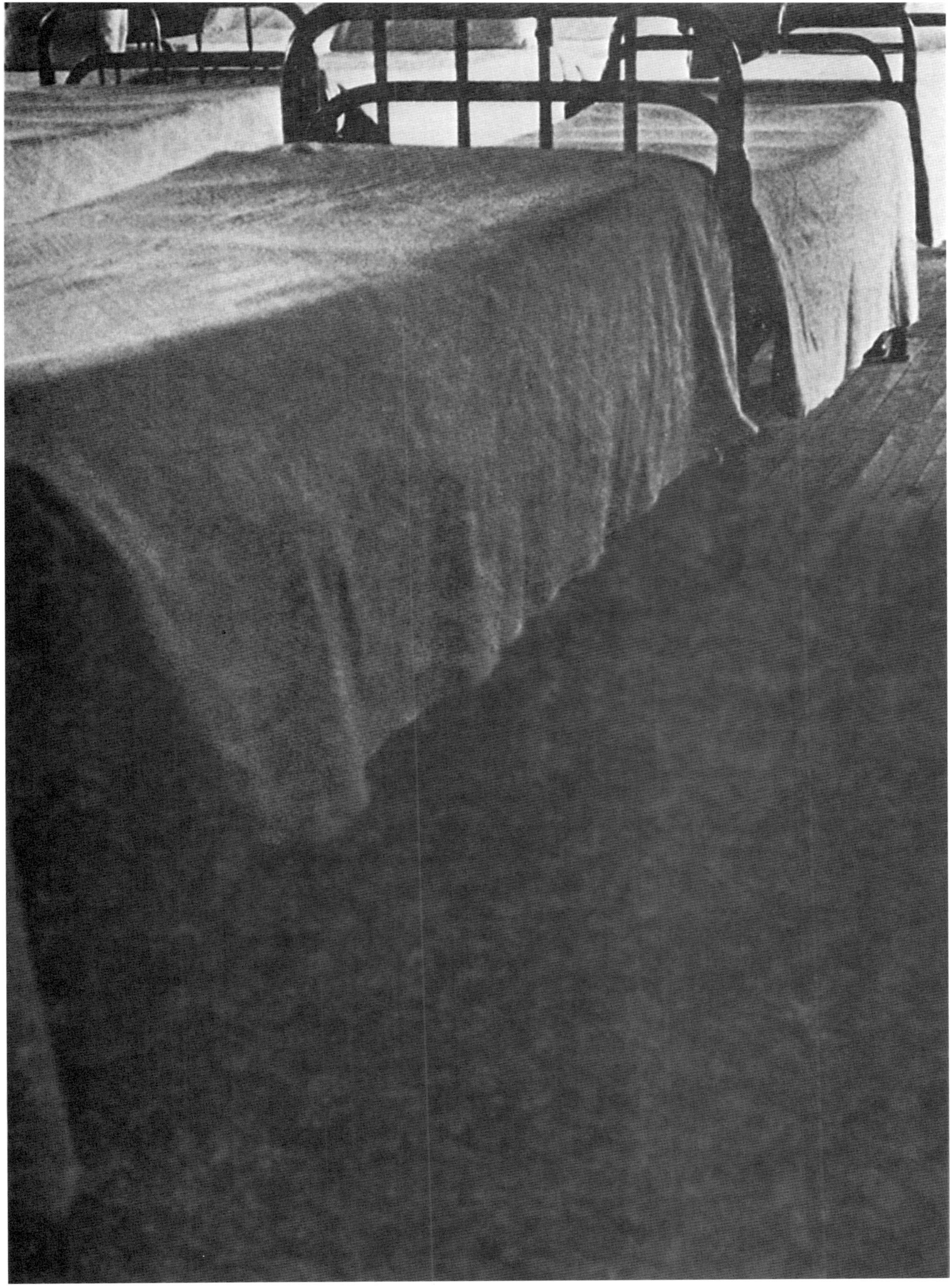

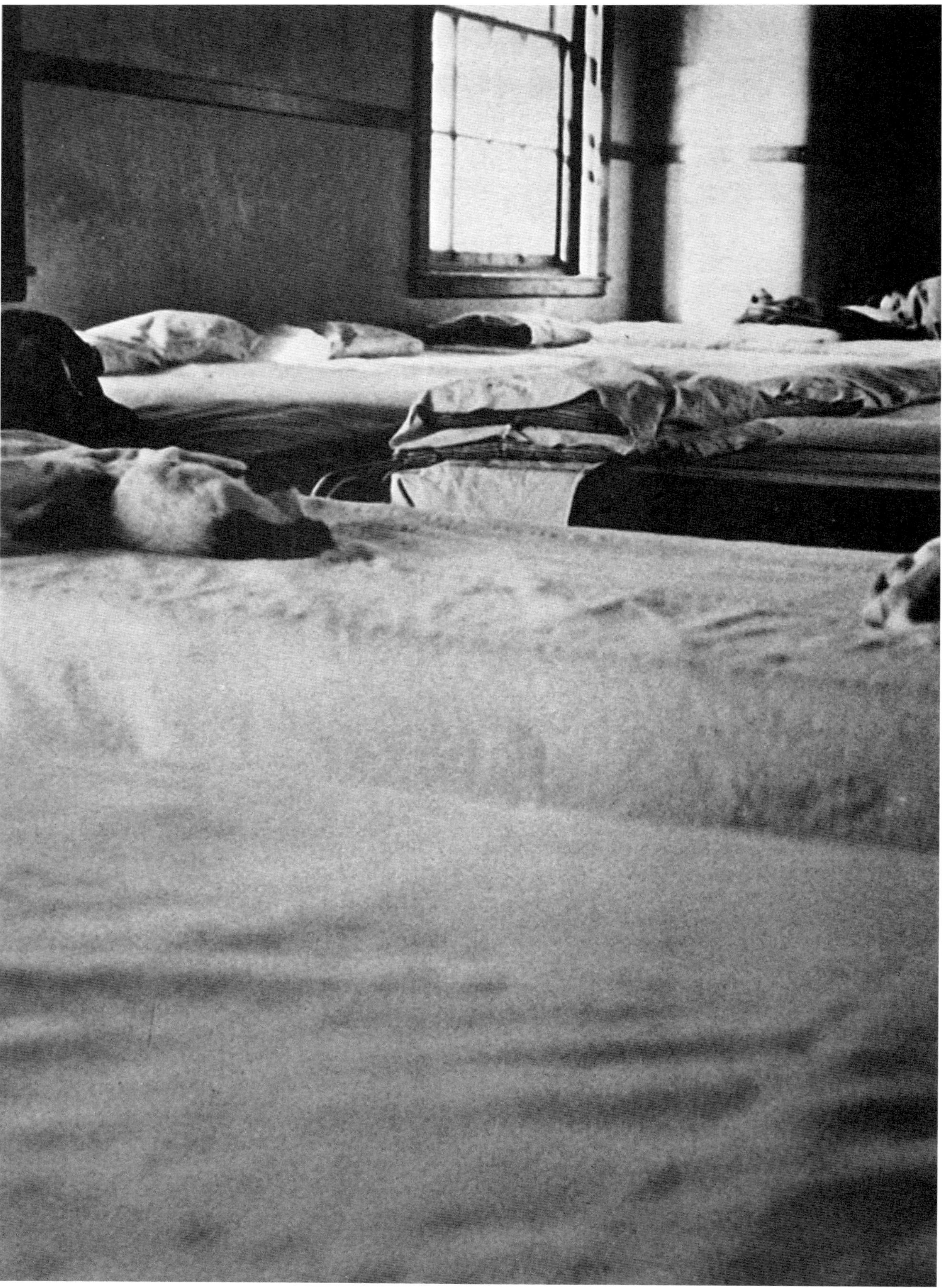

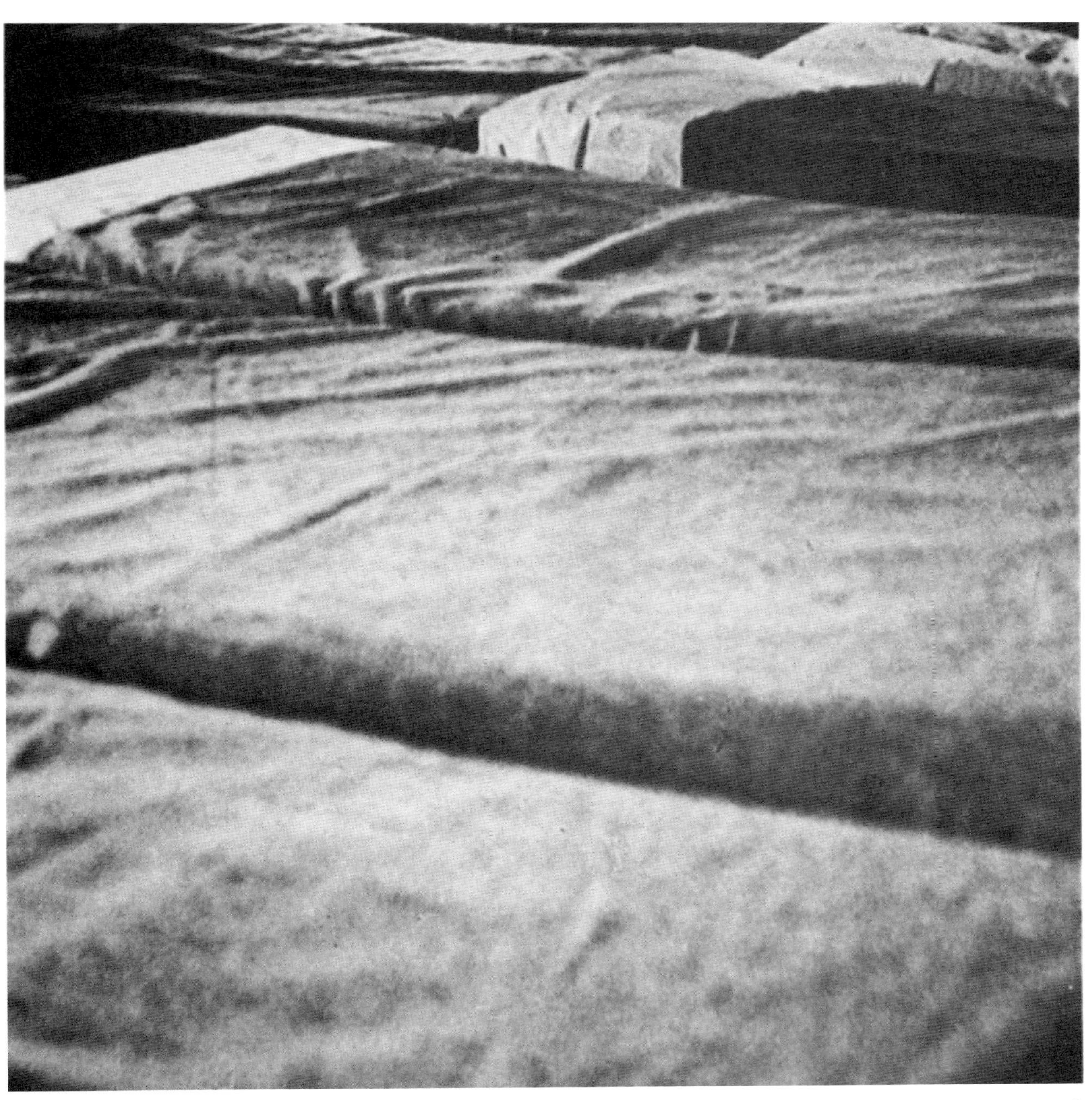

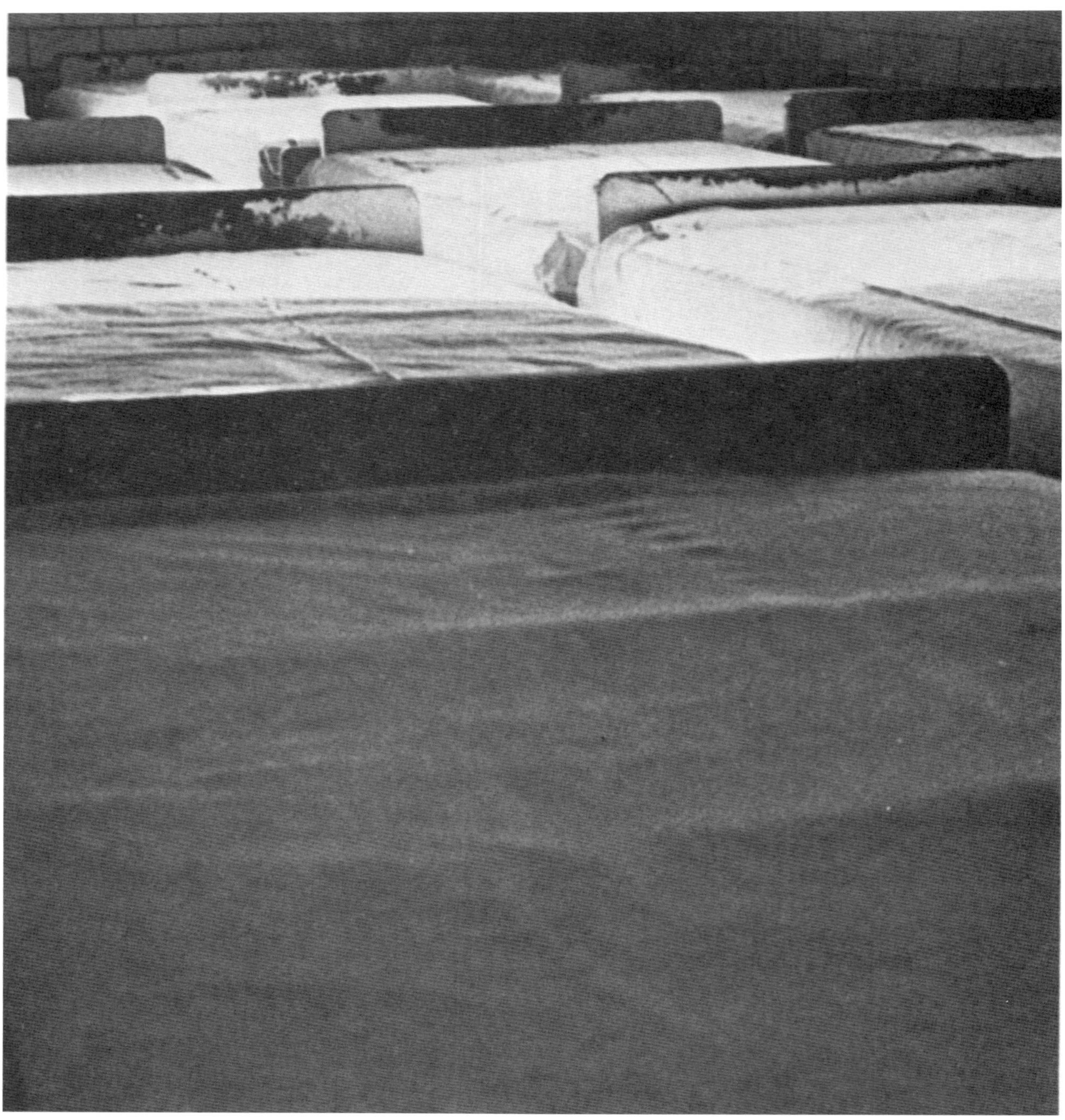

"The limited resources of the State institutions have been taxed beyond the breaking point."

John Fitzgerald Kennedy

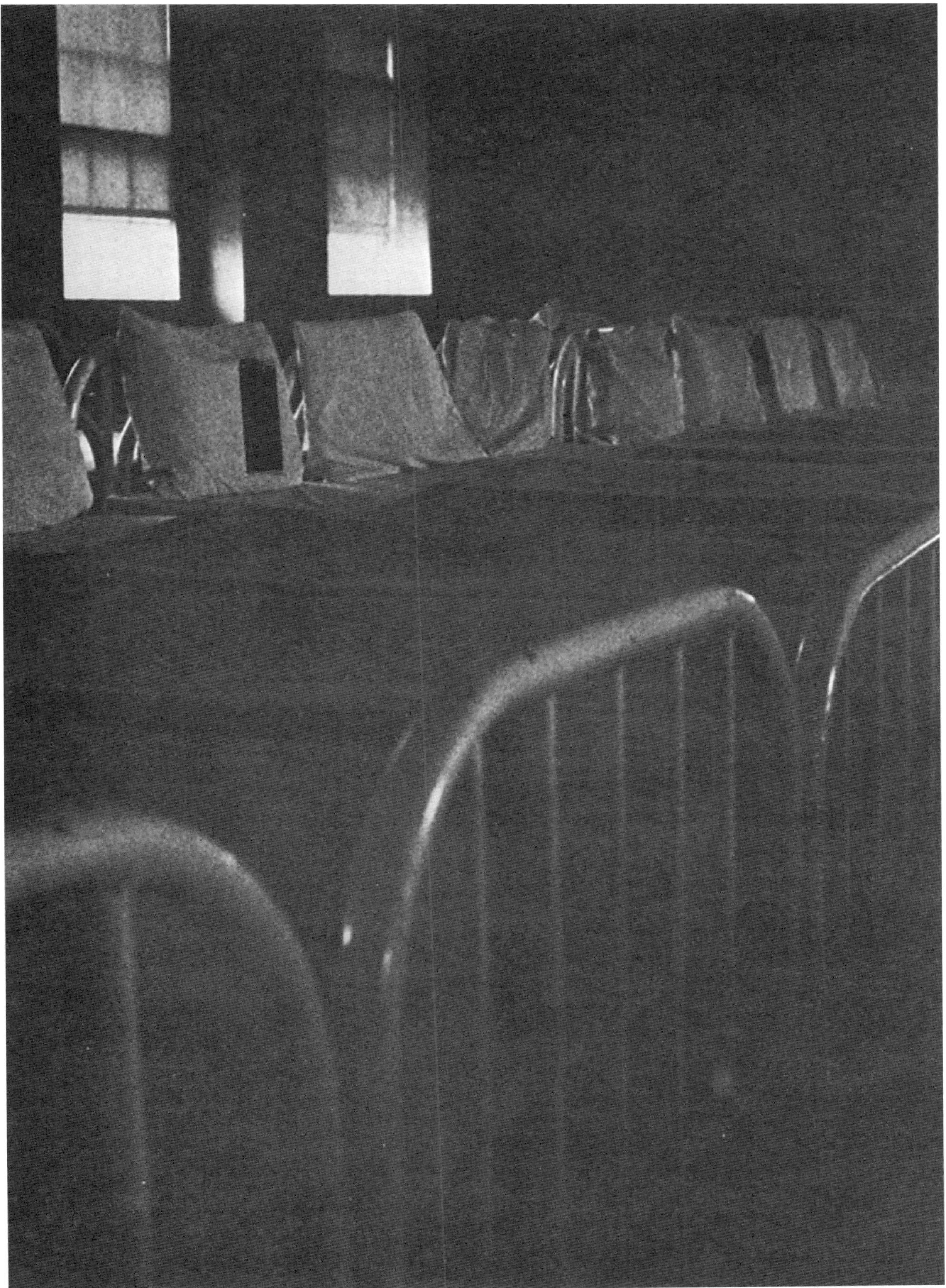

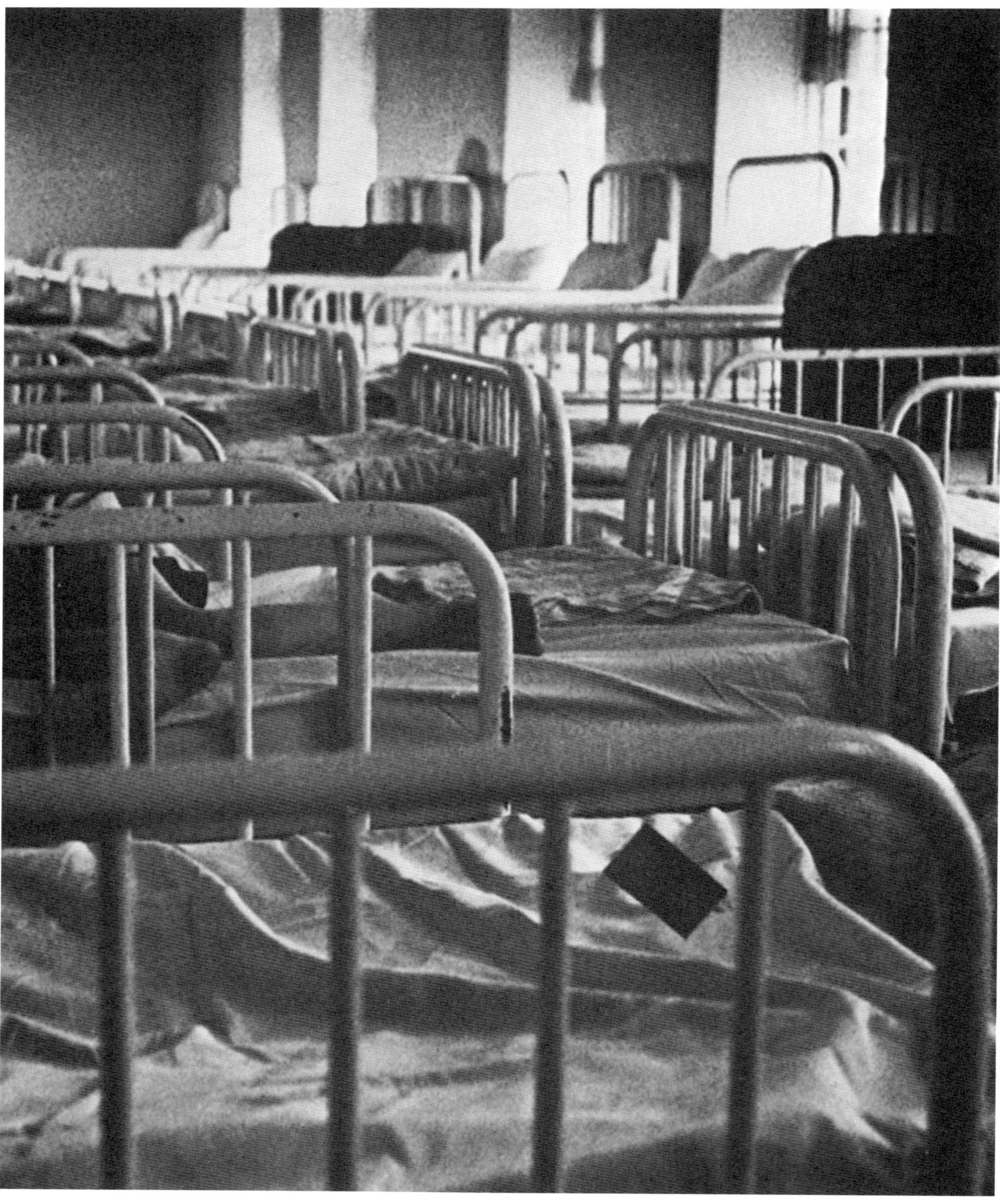

"The quality of care furnished by State institutions varies widely, but from the standpoint of well-qualified and adequate personnel and the availability and use of professional services and modern, progressive programs, the general level must be regarded as low. In large State institutions the normal problems of administration and care are compounded by overcrowding, staff shortages, and frequently by inadequate budgets."

The President's Panel on
Mental Retardation

# "Man's inhumanity to man..."

"Man's inhumanity to man
Makes countless thousands mourn."

Robert Burns

All doors in the living quarters of institutions that we visited had locks, regardless of the age or severity of retardation of the patients immured. These locks are on outside doors as well as inside doors. Doors are made of heavy gauge metal or thick wood. It is routine for attendants to pass from room to room with key chain in hand, unlocking and locking doors en route.

Many dormitories for the severely and moderately retarded ambulatory residents have solitary confinement cells or, what is officially referred to as "thera- peutic isolation." "Therapeutic isolation" means solitary confinement—in its most punitive and inhumane form. These cells are usually located in the basements of large dormitory buildings. Sometimes they are located on an upper floor, off to the side and away from the casual or official visitor's scrutiny. They are generally tiny rooms, approximately seven feet by seven feet, shielded from the outside with a very heavy metal door having either a fine strong screen or metal bars for observation of the "prisoner." Some cells have mattresses, others blankets, still others bare floors. None that we had seen (and we found these cells in each institution visited) had either a bed, a washstand, or a toilet. What we did find in one cell was a thirteen or fourteen year old boy, nude, in a corner of a starkly bare room, lying in his own urine and feces. The boy had been in solitary confinement for several days for committing a minor institutional infraction. Another child, in another institution, had been in solitary confinement for approximately five days for breaking windows. Another had been in isolation through a long holiday weekend because he had struck an attendant. Ironically, in the dormitory where this boy was being incarcerated, we saw another young man who had been "sent to bed early" because he had bitten off the ear of another patient. Apparently, it is infinitely more serious to strike an attendant (and it should not be misunderstood that we condone this) than to bite off the ear of another patient.

In another institution we saw a young man who was glaring at us through the opening in the door of his solitary cell, feces splattered around this opening. He, too, was being punished for breaking an institutional regulation. In this particular dormitory, we had a good opportunity to interview the attendant in charge. We asked him what he needed most in order to better supervise the residents and provide them with a more adequate program. The attendant's major request was for the addition of two more solitary confinement cells, to be built adjacent to the existing two cells that, we were told, were always occupied around the clock, day in and day out.

We saw children with hands tied and legs bound. After discussions with attendants and supervisors in the four institutions, we were convinced that one of the major reasons for the heavy use of solitary confinement and physical restraints was the extraordinary shortage of staff in practically all of these dormitories. The attendant who requested the construction of two additional solitary confinement cells was, with one assistant, responsible for the supervision of an old multilevel dormitory, housing over 100 severely retarded ambulatory adults. Almost in desperation he asked us, "What can one do with those patients who do not conform? We must lock them up, or restrain them, or sedate them, or put fear into them."

At that point, we did not feel we had a response that would satisfy either him or us.

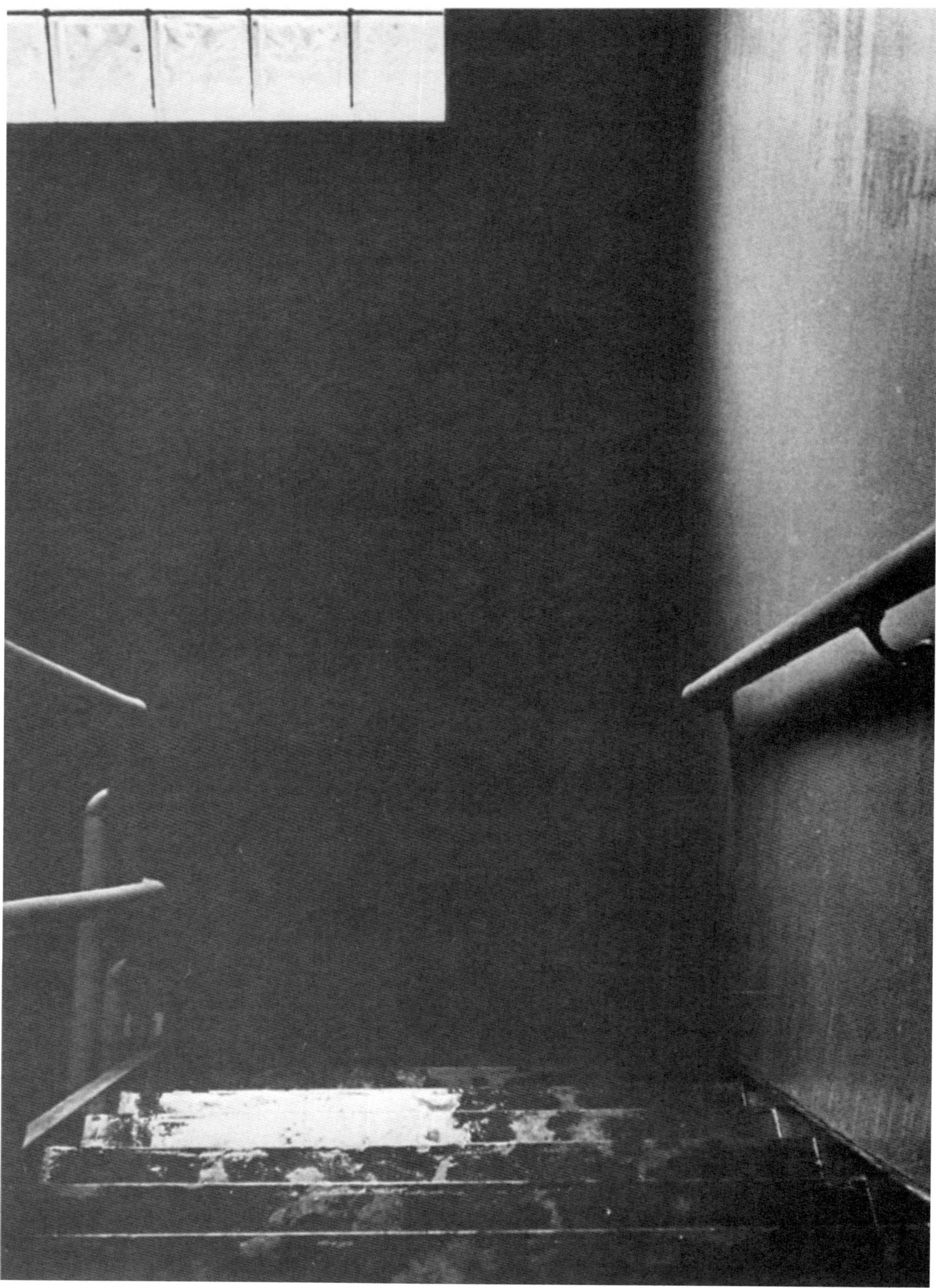

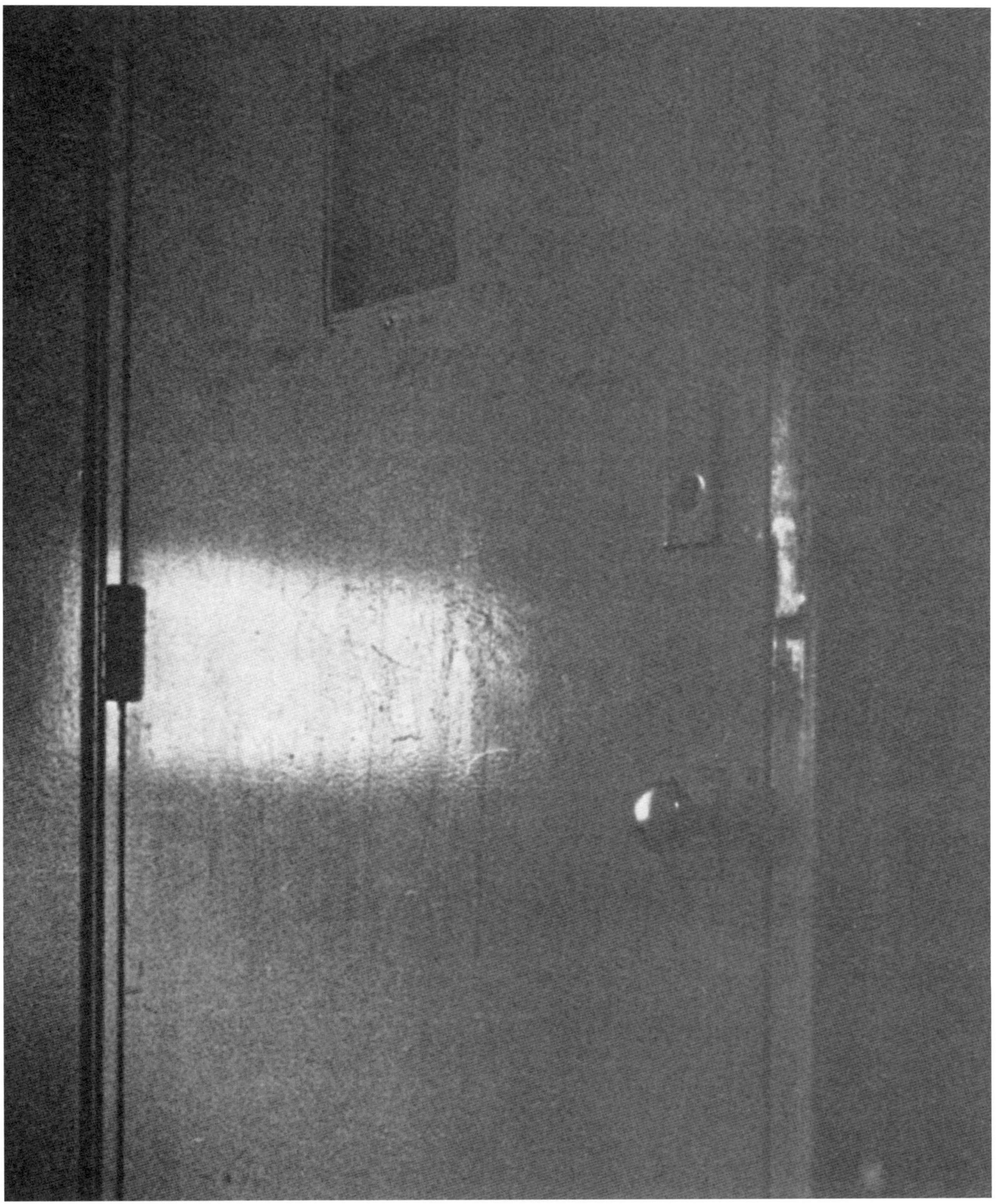

"The door of Death is made of gold
That mortal eyes cannot behold."

William Blake

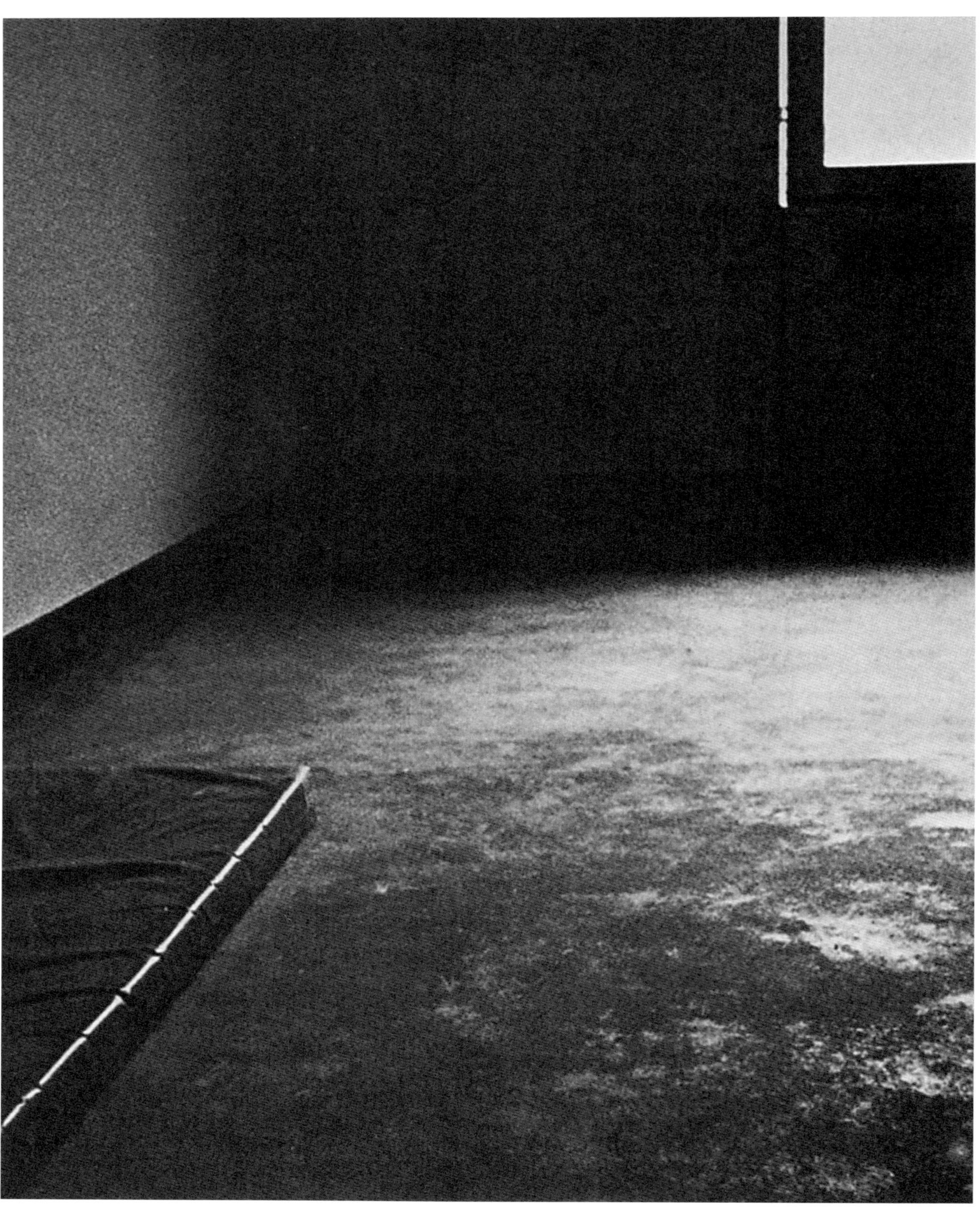
Christmas in Purgatory

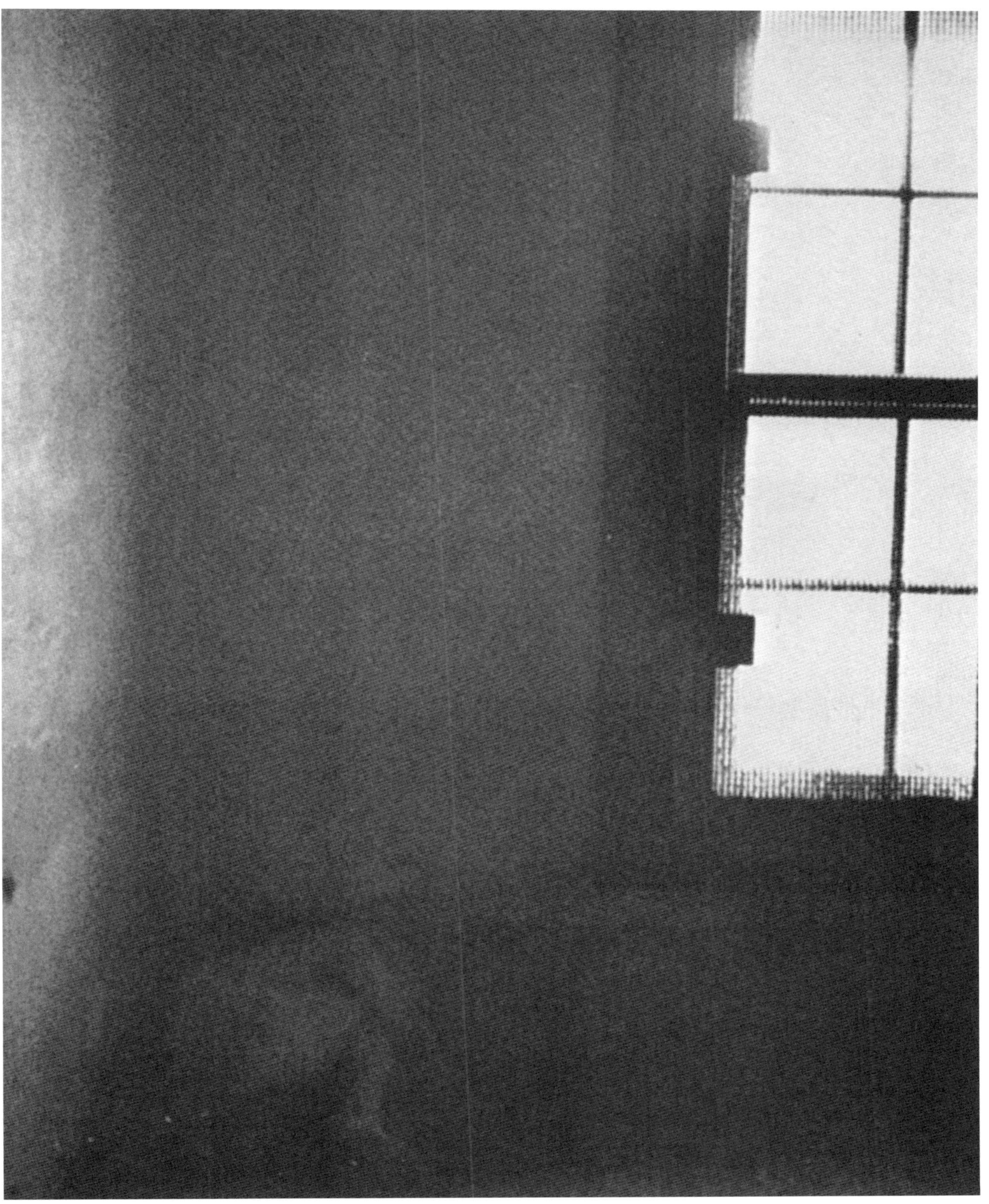

"Inasmuch as ye have done it unto one of the least of
these my brethren, ye have done it unto me."

Matthew, XXV, 40

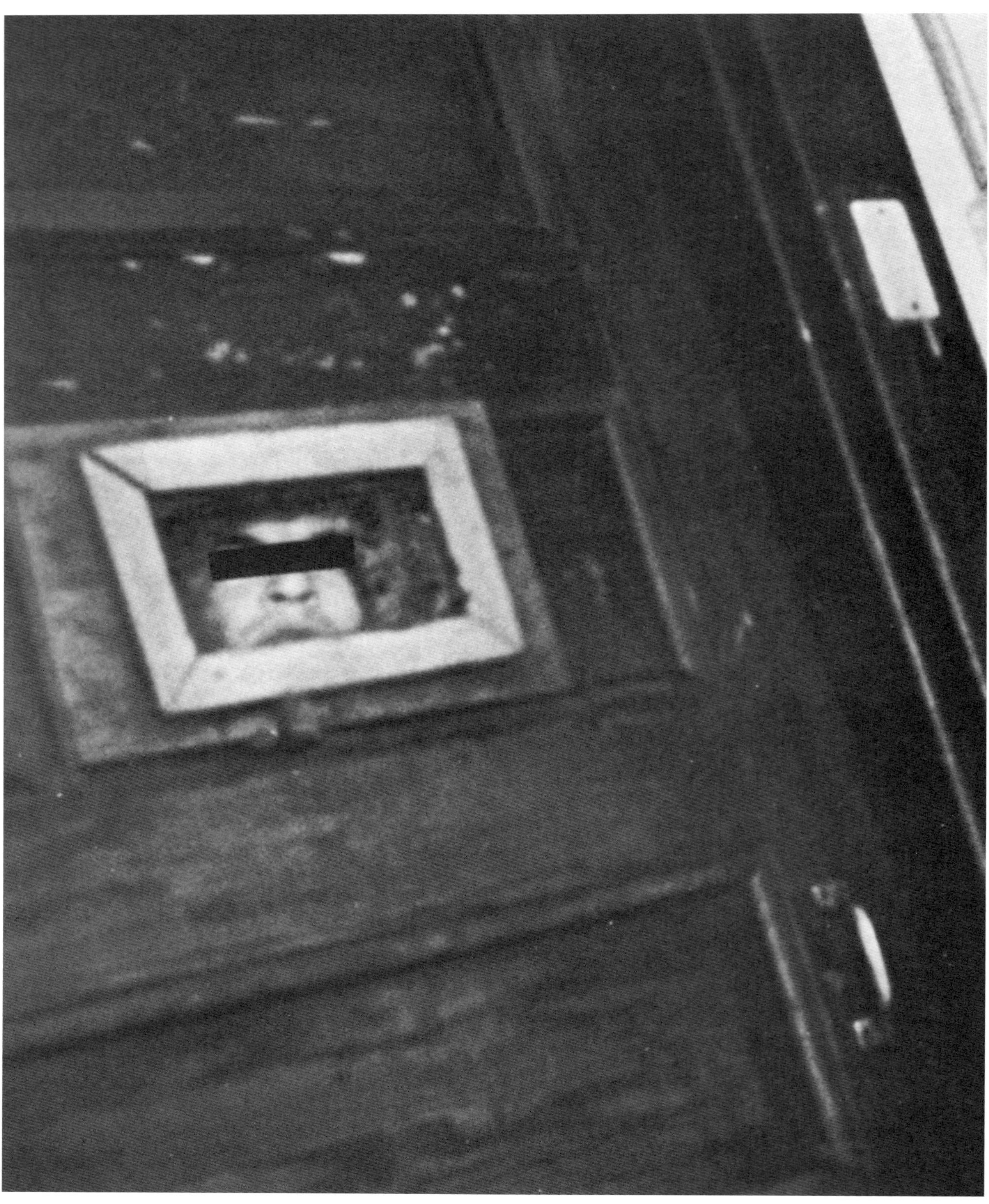

"Some of mankind's most terrible misdeeds have
been committed under the spell of certain magic
words or phrases."

James Bryant Conant

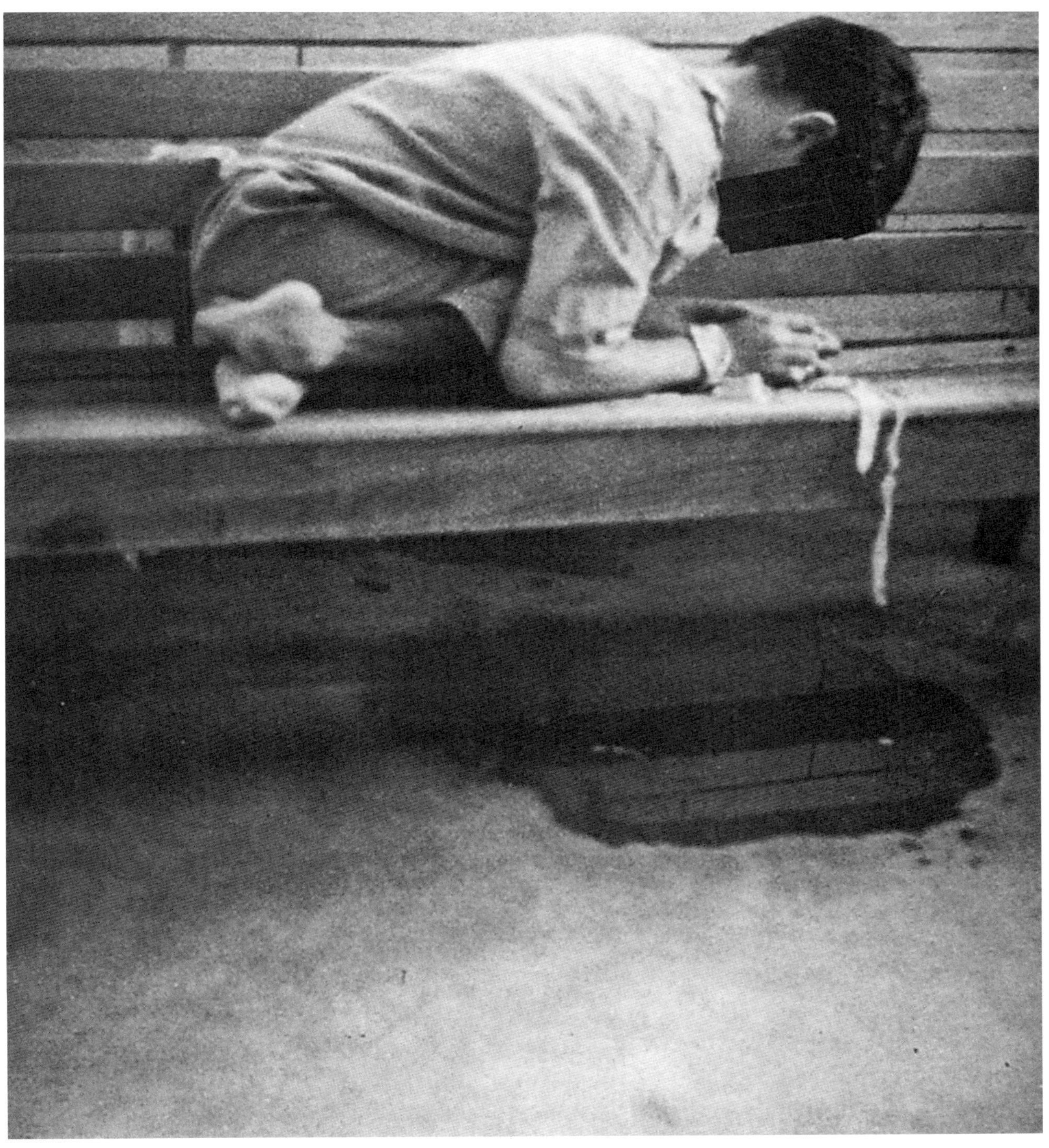

"Oh! why does the wind blow upon me so wild?
Is it because I'm nobody's child?"

Phila Henrietta Case

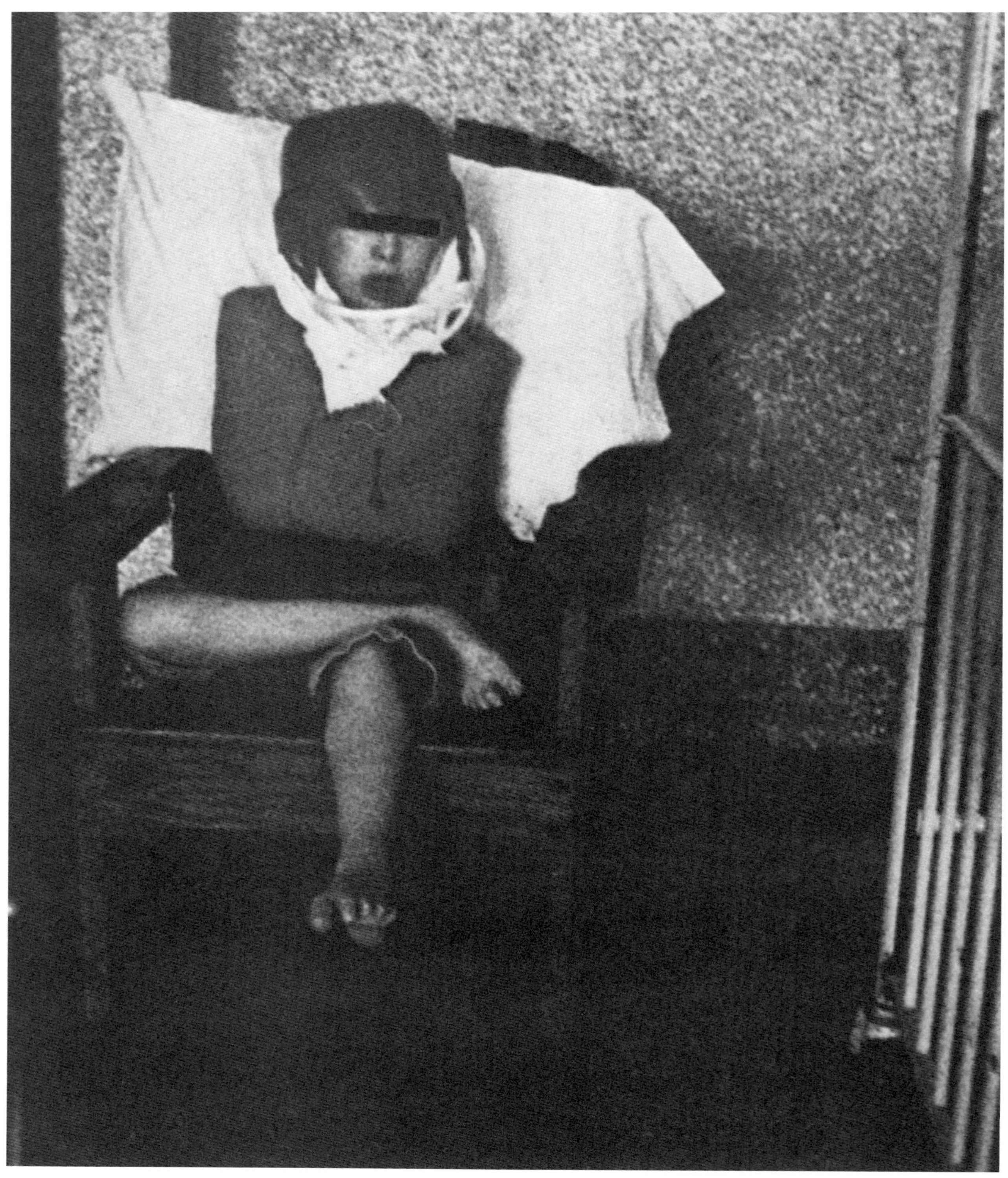

"Perfected and modified according to circumstance, chains gave way (during the early nineteenth century) to a long series of other ingenuous contrivances, all designed to limit the patient's freedom of movement. According to Oegg, restraining devices were generally thought to be as necessary for the preservation of life as eating, drinking, etc."

Emil Kraepelin

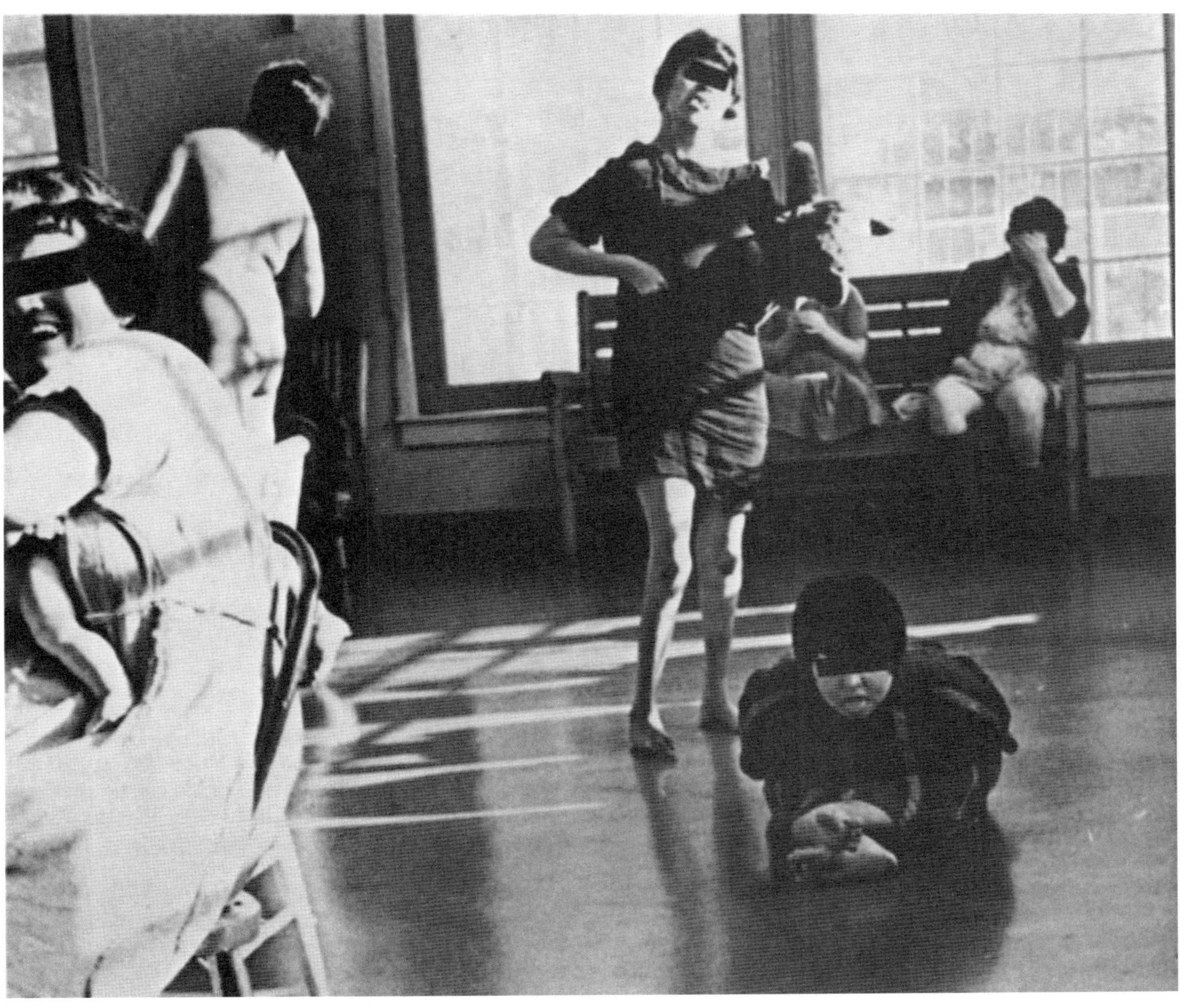

# "I sometimes wish that God were back..."

"I sometimes wish that God were back
In this dark world and wide;
For though some virtues he might lack,
He had his pleasant side."

Gamaliel Bradford

In each of the dormitories for severely retarded residents, there is what is euphemistically called a day room or recreation room. The odor in each of these rooms is overpowering. After a visit to a day room we had to send our clothes to the dry cleaners to have the stench removed. The facilities often contribute to the horror. Floors are sometimes wooden and excretions are rubbed into the cracks, leaving permanent stench. Most day rooms have a series of bleacher benches, on which sit unclad residents, jammed together, without purposeful activity, communication, or any interaction. In each day room is an attendant or two, whose main function seems to be to "stand around" and, on occasion, hose down the floor "driving" excretions into a sewer conveniently located in the center of the room.

We were invited into female as well as male day rooms, in spite of the supervisor's knowledge that we, male visitors, would be observ-ing naked females. In one such dormitory, with an overwhelming odor, we noticed feces on the wooden ceilings, and on the patients as well as the floors.

The question one might ask is, Is it possible to prevent these conditions? Although we are convinced that to teach severely retarded adults to wear clothes one must invest time and patience, we believe it is possible to do so—given adequate staff. There is one more requirement. The staff has to be convinced that residents <u>can</u> be taught to wear clothes, that they <u>can</u> be engaged in purposeful activities, that they <u>can</u> learn to control their bladders. The staff has to believe that their "boys" and "girls" are human beings who can learn. Obviously, the money and the additional staff are vitally important. However, even more important, is the fundamental belief that each of these residents is a human being.

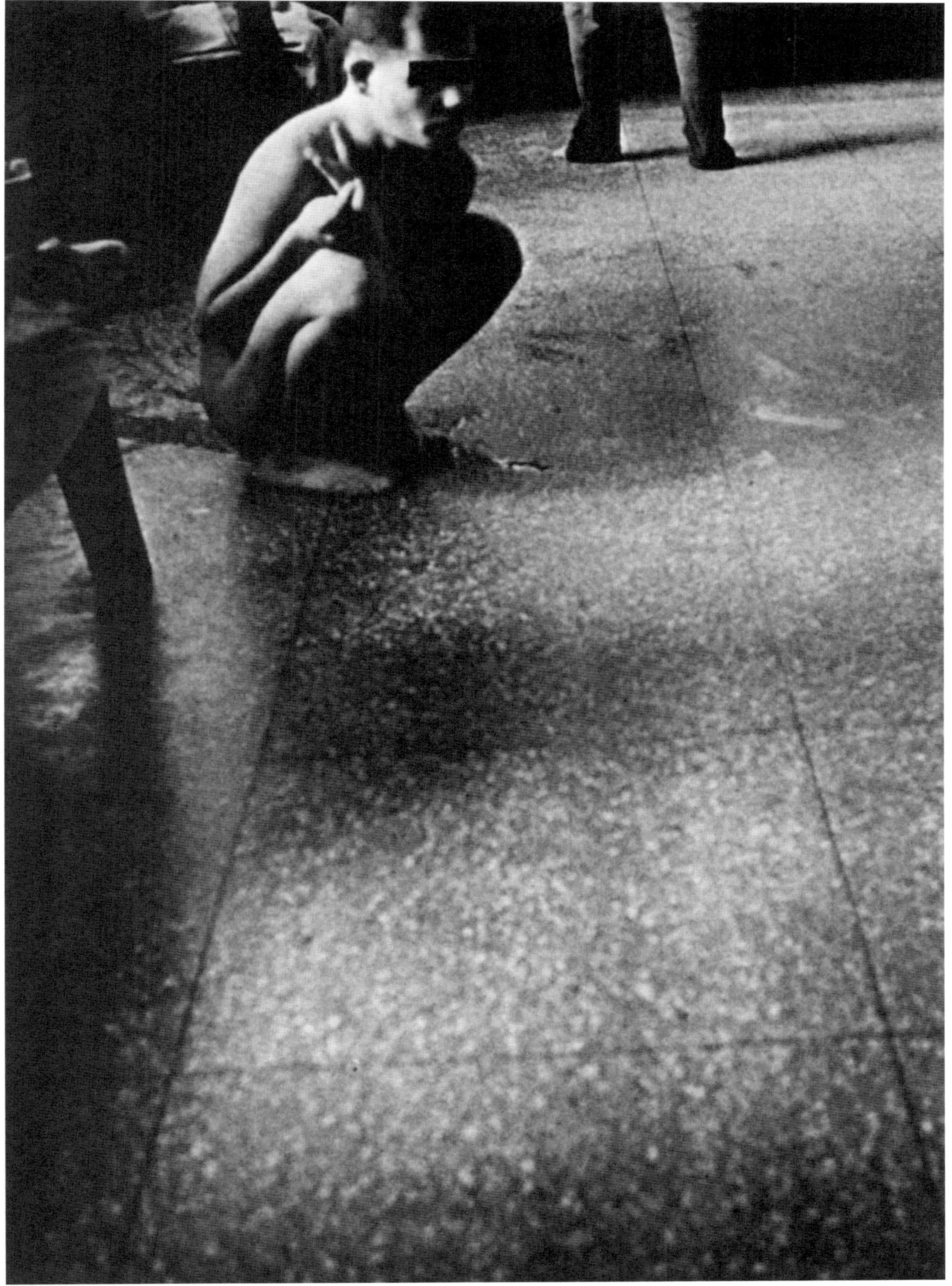

# Christmas in Purgatory

"He is never less at leisure than when at leisure."

Cicero

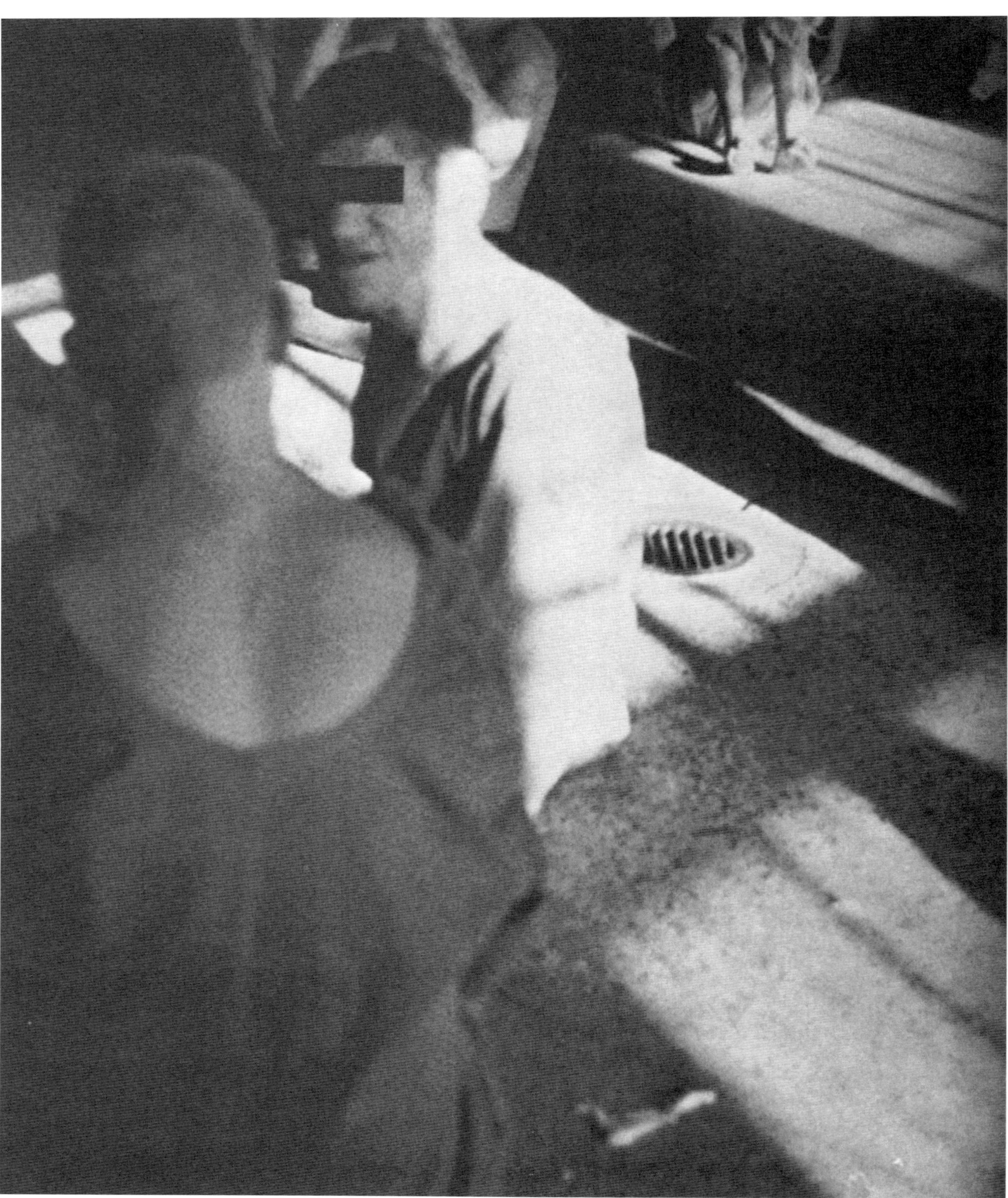

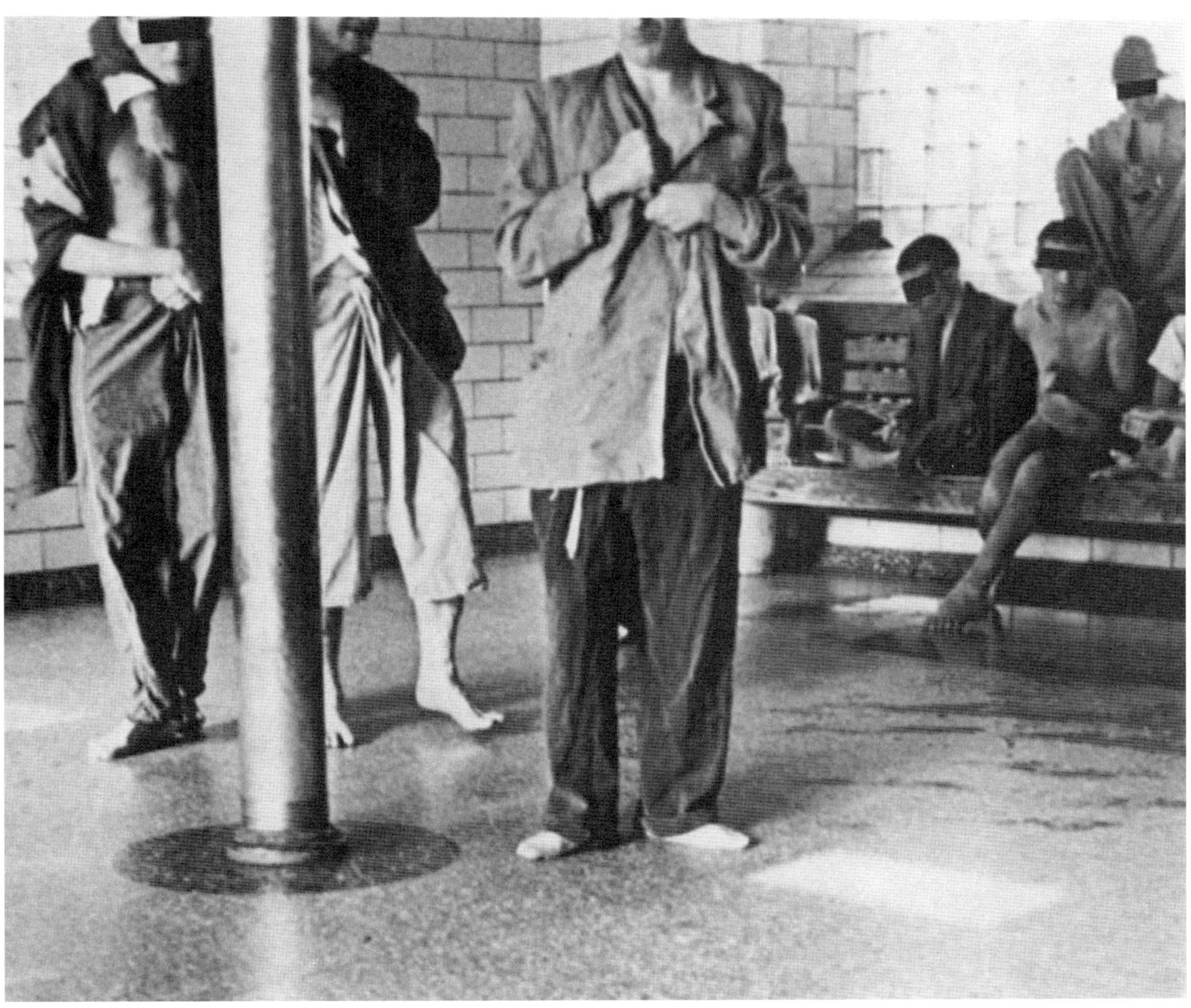

"Thank heaven! The crisis—
The danger is passed,
And the lingering illness
Is over at last—
And the fever called 'Living'
Is conquered at last."

Edgar Allen Poe

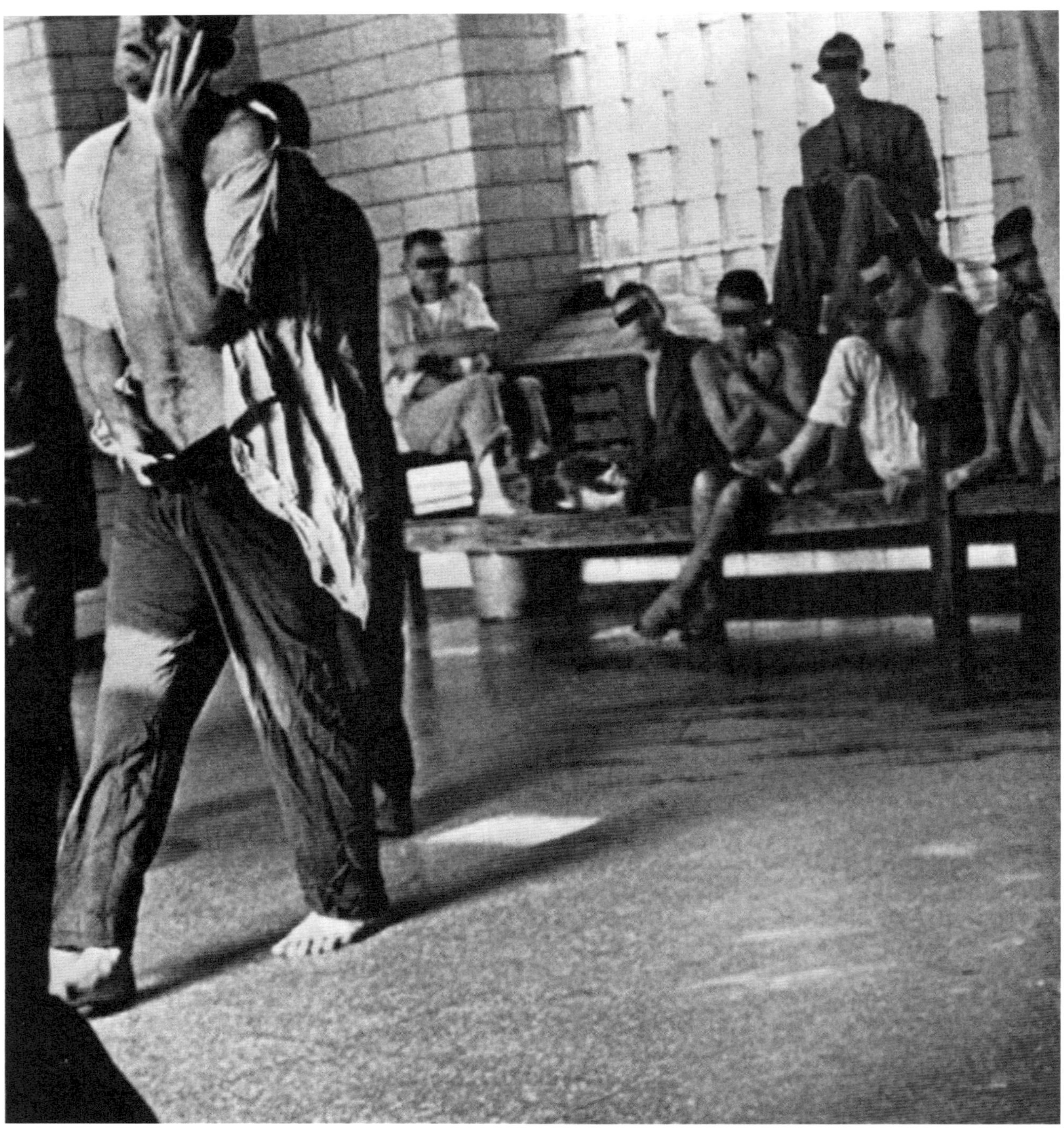

"Stupid or mentally deficient patients (during the early nineteen century) because they seemed passively to endure whatever was inflicted upon them, gave rise to the popular assumption that they were insensitive to hunger, cold, and pain even though the opposite was proven by their obvious emaciation, by their frozen members, and by their dying from injuries. The result was that their suffering was looked upon as self-evident and unalterable while the significance of their plight was never fully appreciated."

Emil Kraepelin

26

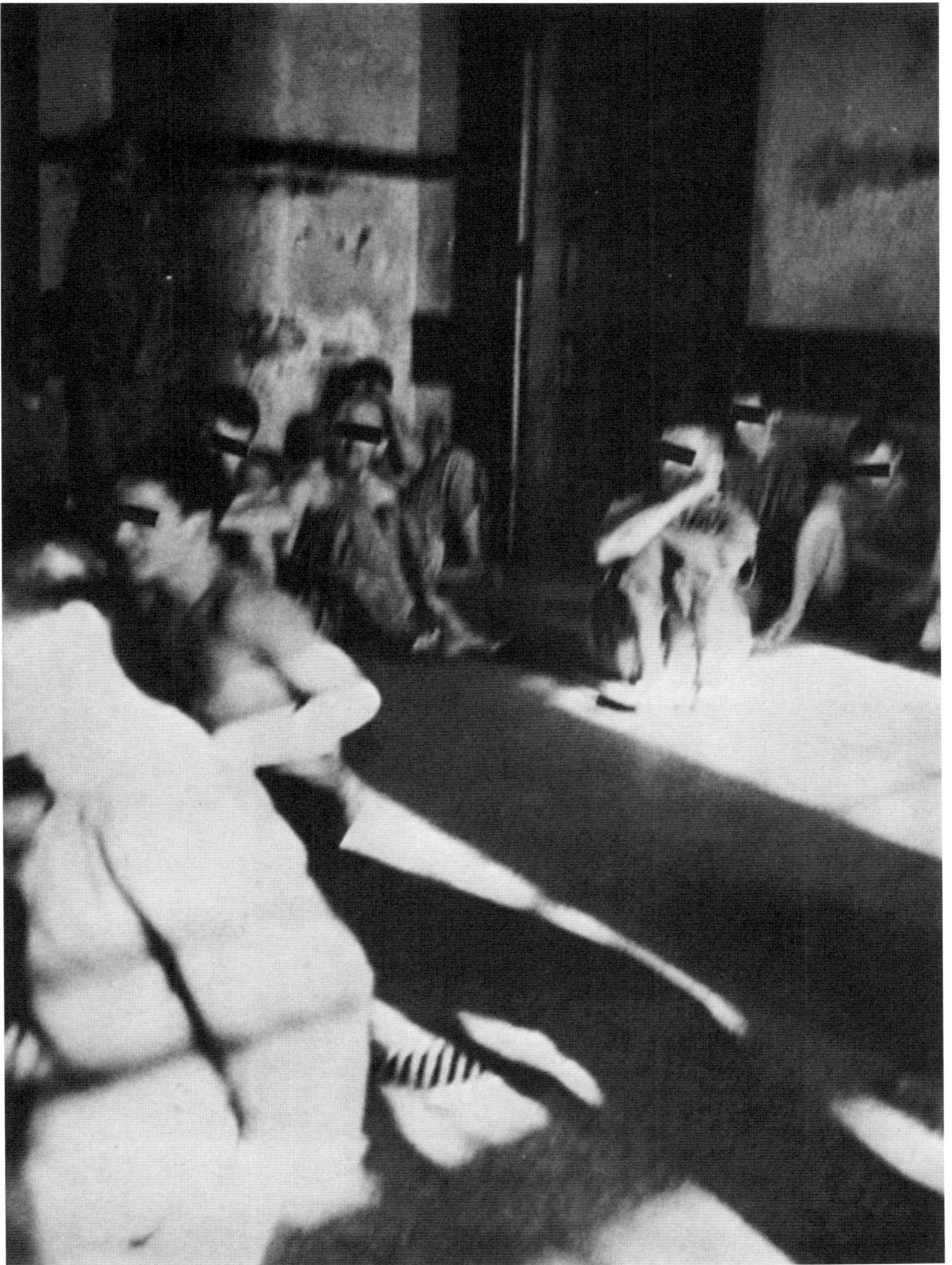

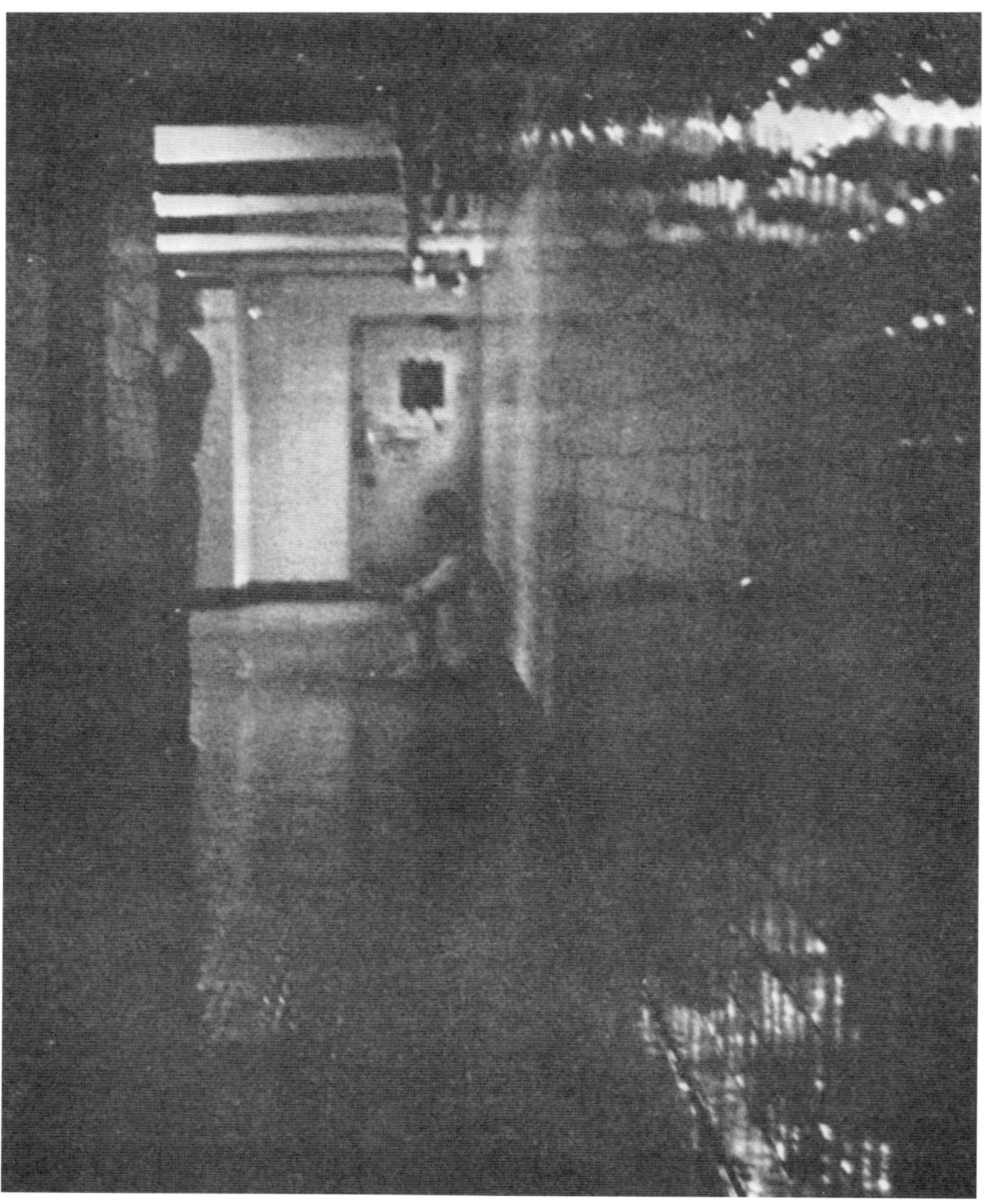

"You shall not wrong a stranger or oppress him,
for you were strangers in the land of Egypt."

Exodus, 23:5

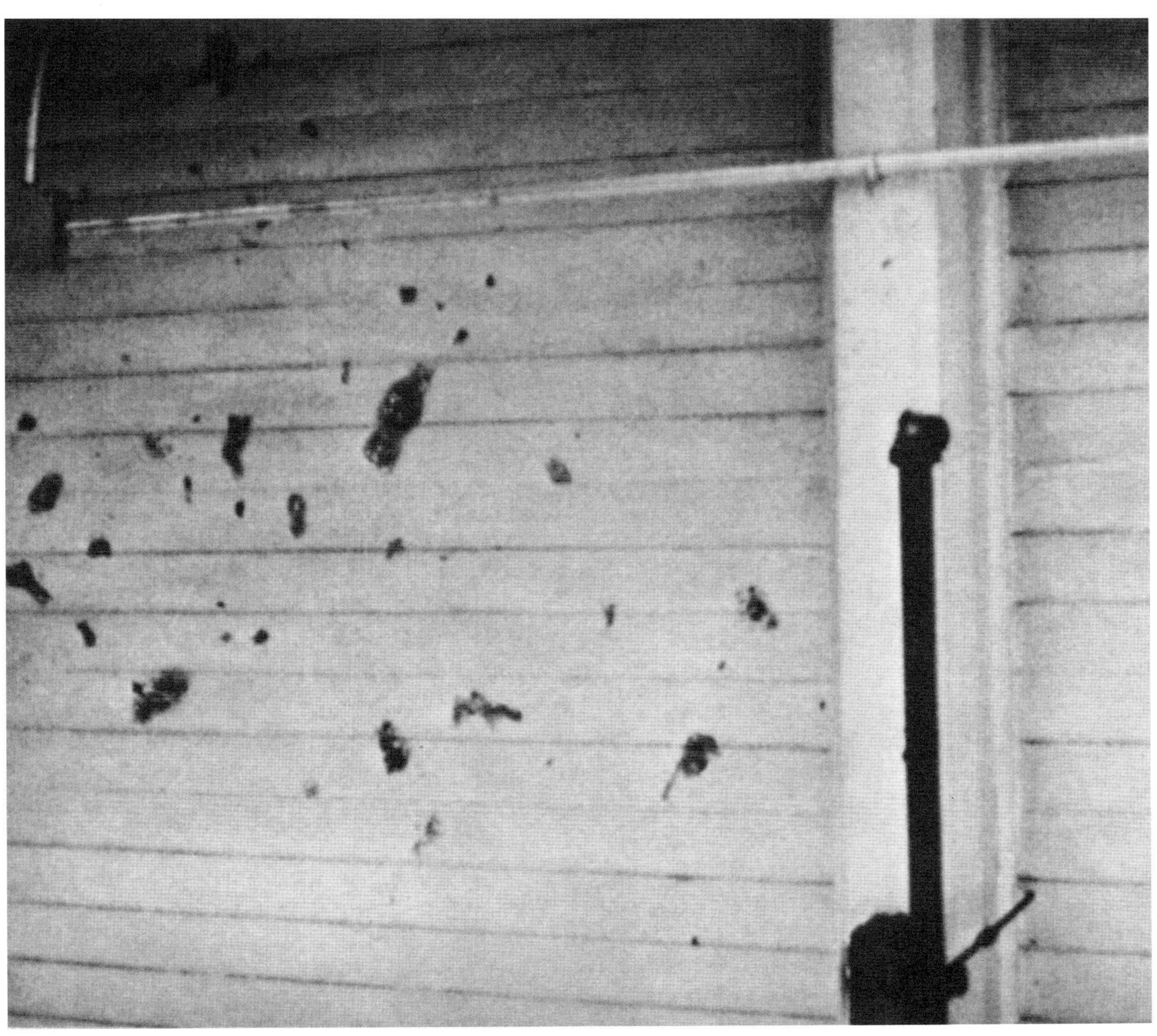

"A humanitarian is bound to shudder when he discovers the plight of the unfortunate victims of this dreadful affliction; many of them grovel in their own filth on unclean straw that is seldom changed, often stark naked and in chains, in dark, damp dungeons where no breath of fresh air can enter. Under such terrifying conditions, it would be easier for the most rational person to become insane than for a made man to regain his sanity."

Anonymous, 1795

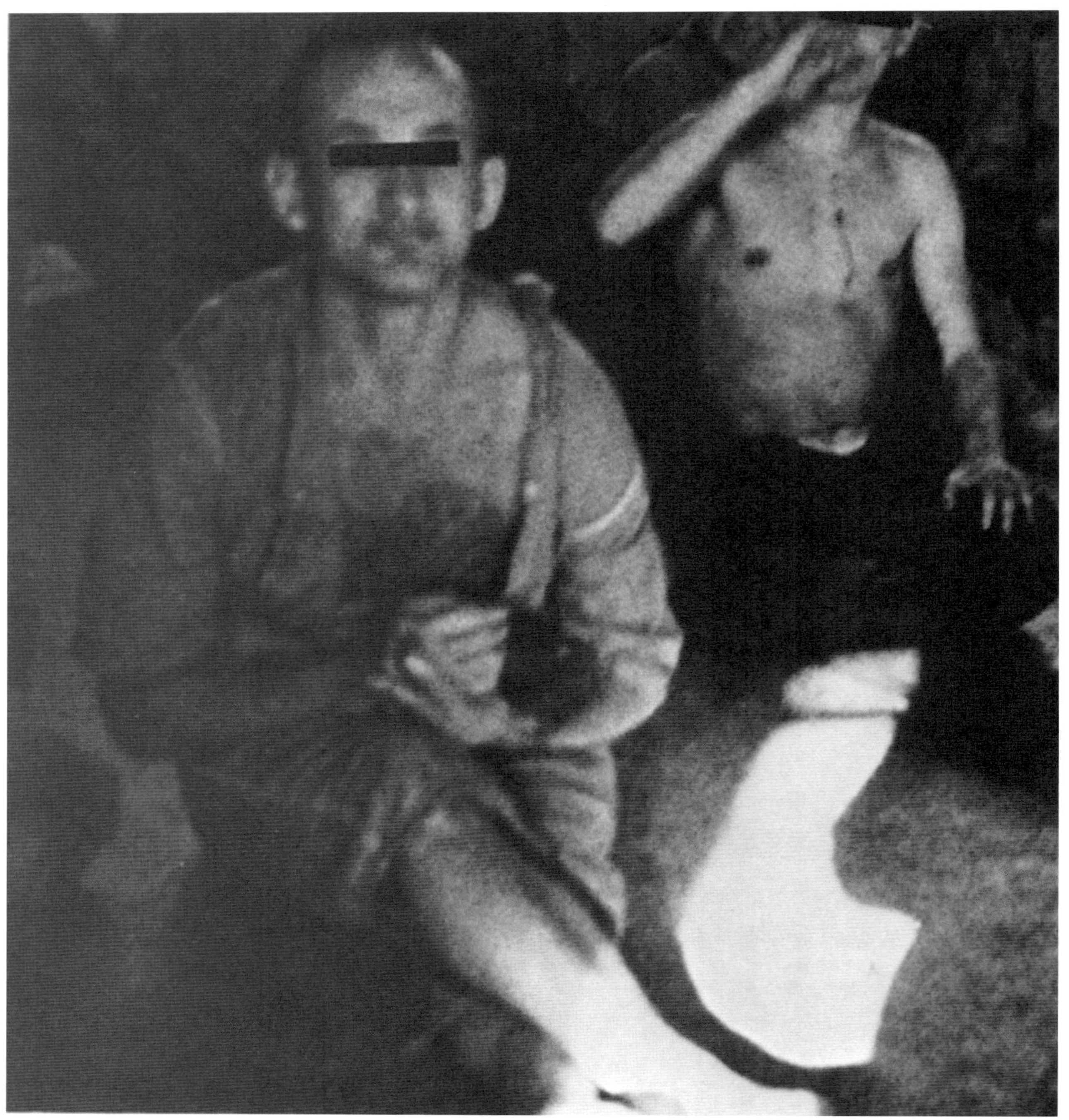

"Am I my brother's keeper?"

Genesis IV, 9

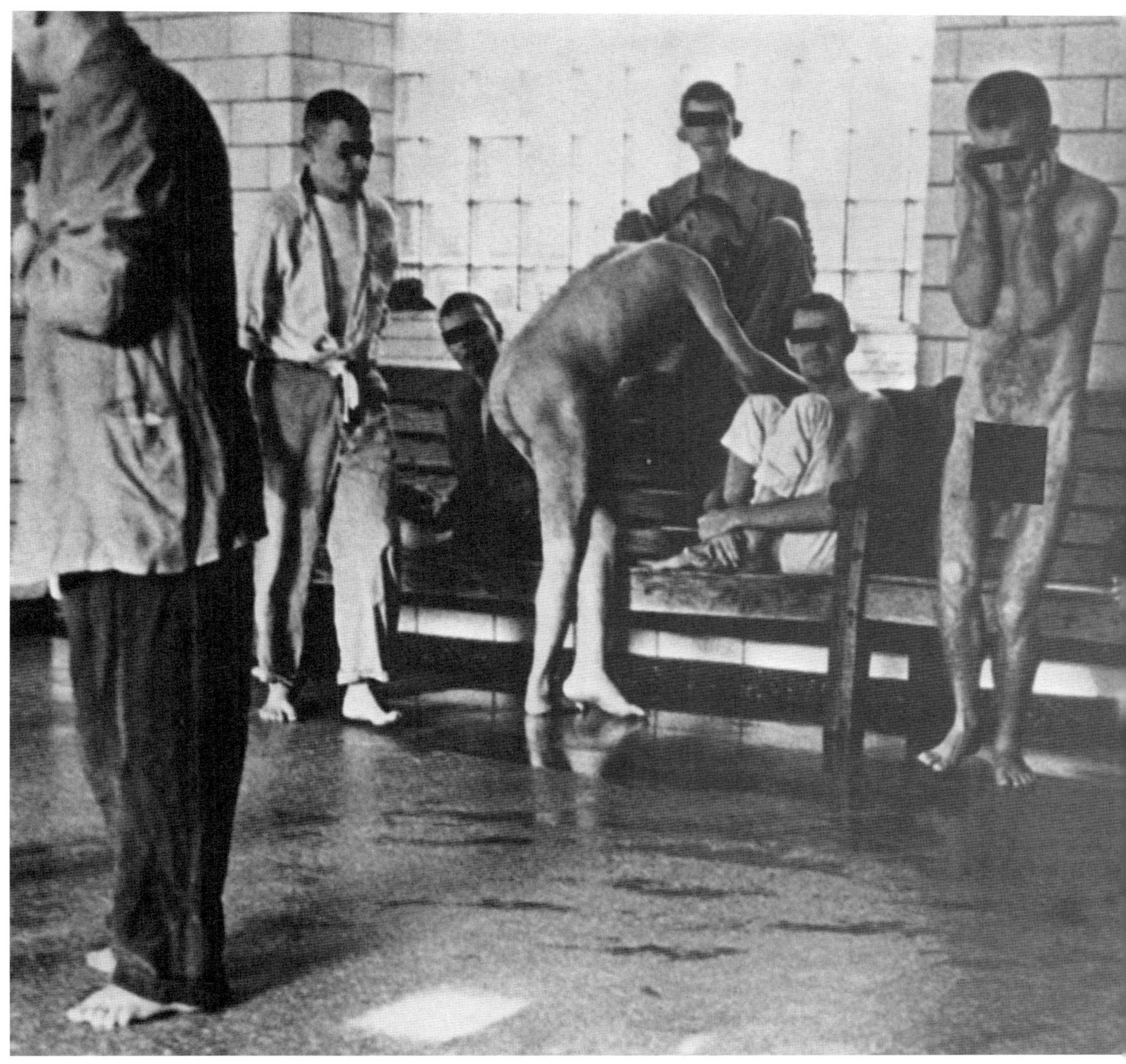

"In the asylum in Berlin those who are stark raving mad are isolated for the duration of their madness; they are locked naked…"

Hoch, 1804

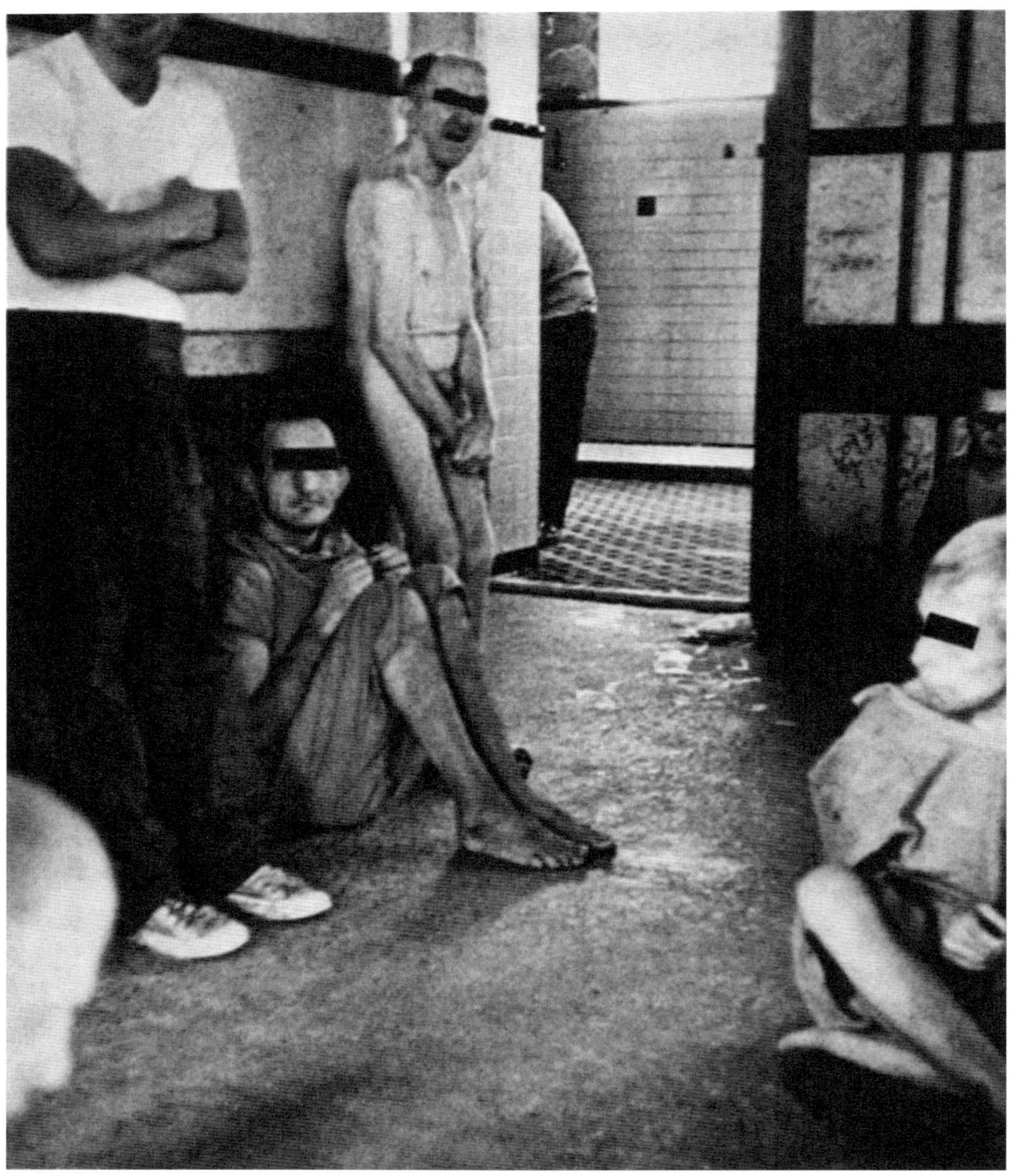

"I saw patients naked, with rags or nothing more than straw to protect them against the cold, damp weather. I saw how in their wretched state they were deprived of fresh air to breathe, of water to quench their thirst, and of the basic necessities of life. I saw them turned over for safe keeping to brutal jailers. I saw them chained in damp, cramped holes without light or air; people would be ashamed to keep in such places the wild animals that are cared for at great expense in our large cities. This is what I observed almost everywhere in France, and that is how the mentally ill are treated almost everywhere in Europe."

Esquirol, 1818

"While the difference between <u>becoming</u> or not becoming mentally subnormal may often be slight, the difference between <u>being</u> and not being mentally subnormal may be considerable."

Albert T. Murphy

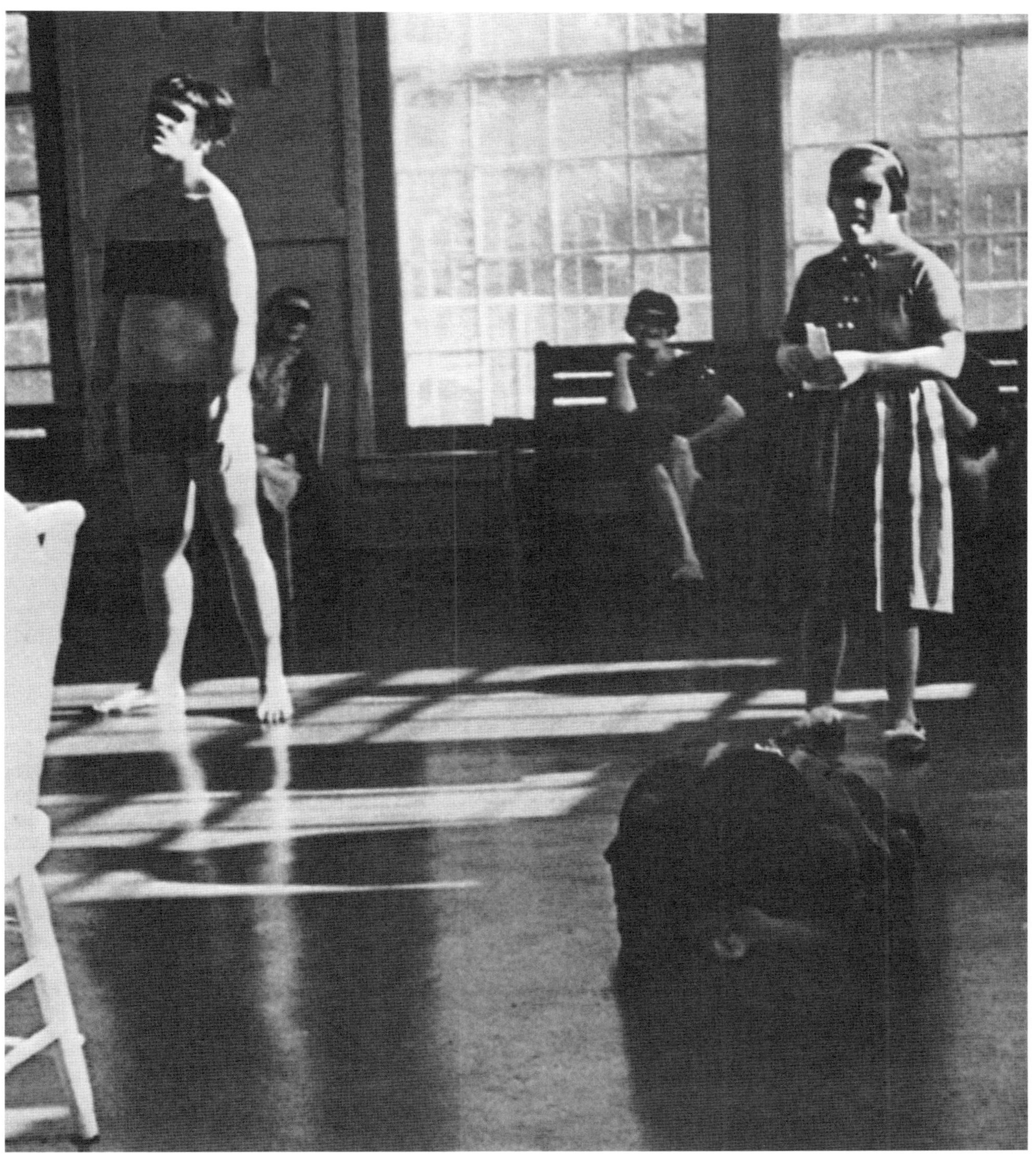

# "Suffer the little children…"

"Suffer the little children…"

The infant dormitories depressed us the most. Here, cribs were placed—as in the other dormitories—side by side and head to head. Very young children, one and two years of age, were lying in cribs, without interaction with any adult, without playthings, without any apparent stimulation. In one dormitory, that had over 100 infants and was connected to 9 other dormitories that totaled 1,000 infants, we experienced a heartbreaking encounter. As we entered, we heard a muffled sound emanating from the "blind" side of a doorway. A young child seemed to be calling, "Come. Come play with me. Touch me." We walked to the door. On the other side were forty or more unkempt infants crawling around a bare floor in a bare room. One of the children had managed to squeeze his hand under the doorway and push his face through the side of the latched door. His moan was the clearest representation we have ever heard of the lonely, hopeless man. In other day rooms, we saw groups of 20 and 30 very young children lying, rocking, sleeping, sitting—alone. Each of these rooms were without toys or adult human contact, although each had desperate looking adult attendants "standing by."

In another dormitory, we were taken on a tour by a chief physician who was anxious to show us a child who had a very rare medical condition. The doctor explained to us that, aside from the child's dwarfism and misshapen body, one of the primary methods for diagnosing this condition is the deep guttural voice. In order to demonstrate this, he pinched the child. The child did not make any sound. He pinched her again, and again—harder, and still harder. Finally, as if in desperation, he insured her response with a pinch that turned into a gouge and caused the child to scream in obvious pain.

In some of the children's dormitories, we observed "nursery programs." What surprised us most was their scarcity and the primitiveness of those in operation. Therefore, we were not unprepared to see several children with severe head lacerations. We were told these were "head bangers." Head banging is another condition that some people think is inevitable when confronted with young severely mentally retarded children. We challenge this. We have reason to believe that head banging can be drastically reduced in an environment where children have other things to do.

The "Special Education" we observed in the dormitories for young children was certainly not education. But, it was special. It was among the most especially frightening and depressing encounters with human beings we have ever experienced.

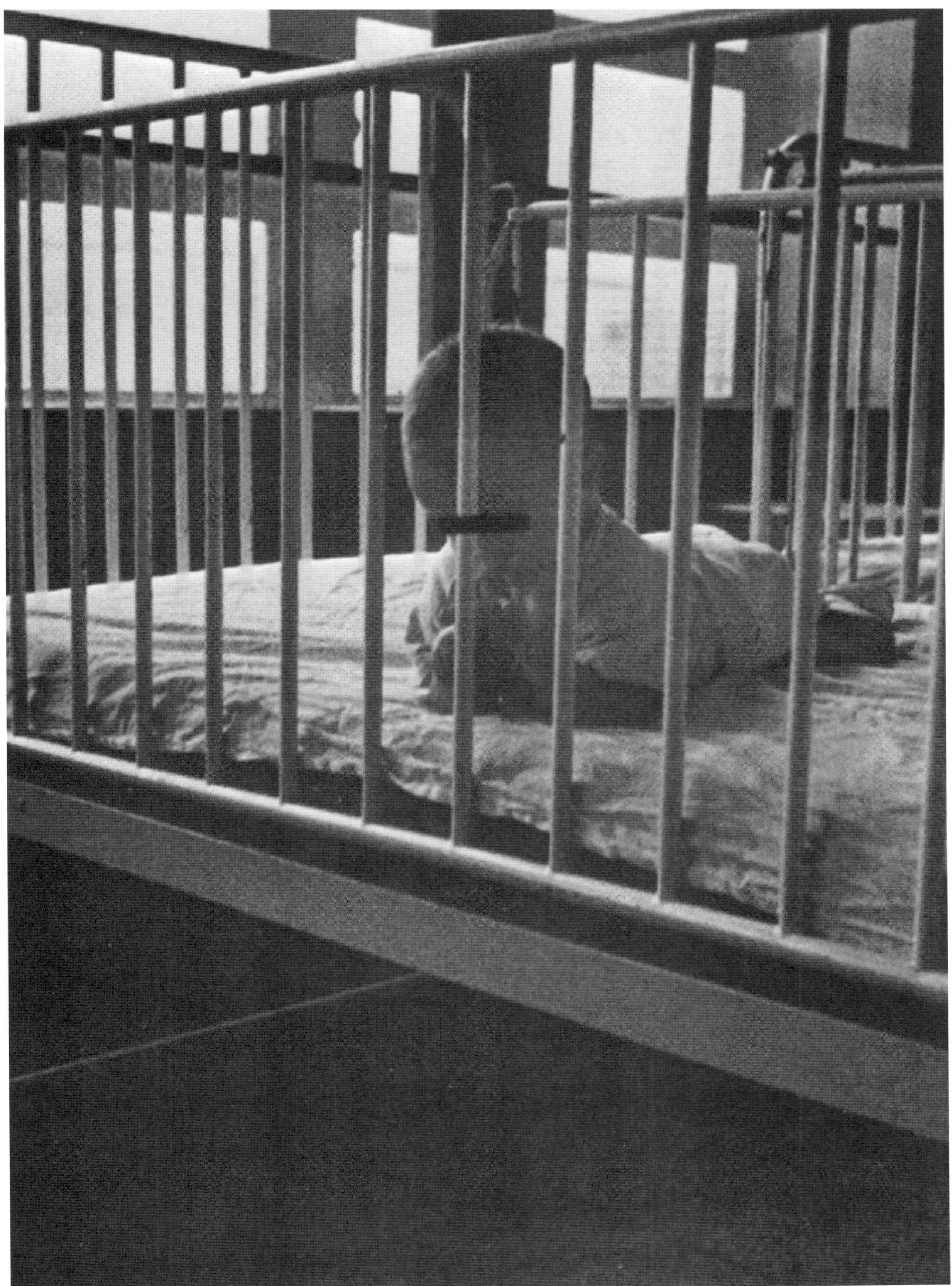

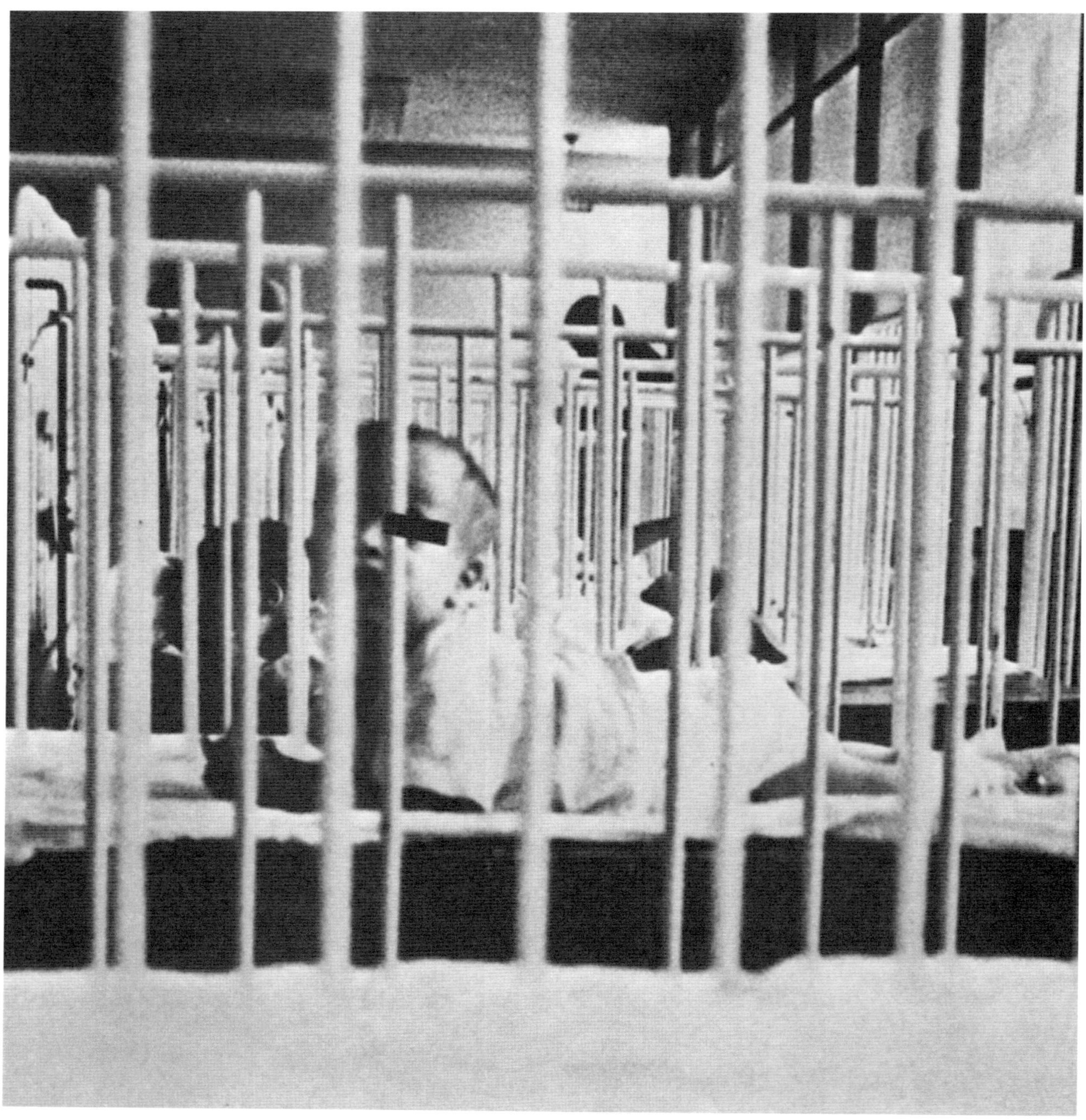

"Cast upon this globe without physical strength or innate ideas, incapable in himself of obeying the fundamental laws of this nature which call him to the supreme place in the universe, it is only in the heart of society that man can attain the pre-eminent position which is his natural destiny. Without the aid of civilization he would be one of the feeblest and least intelligent of animals..."

Jean-Marc-Gaspard Itard

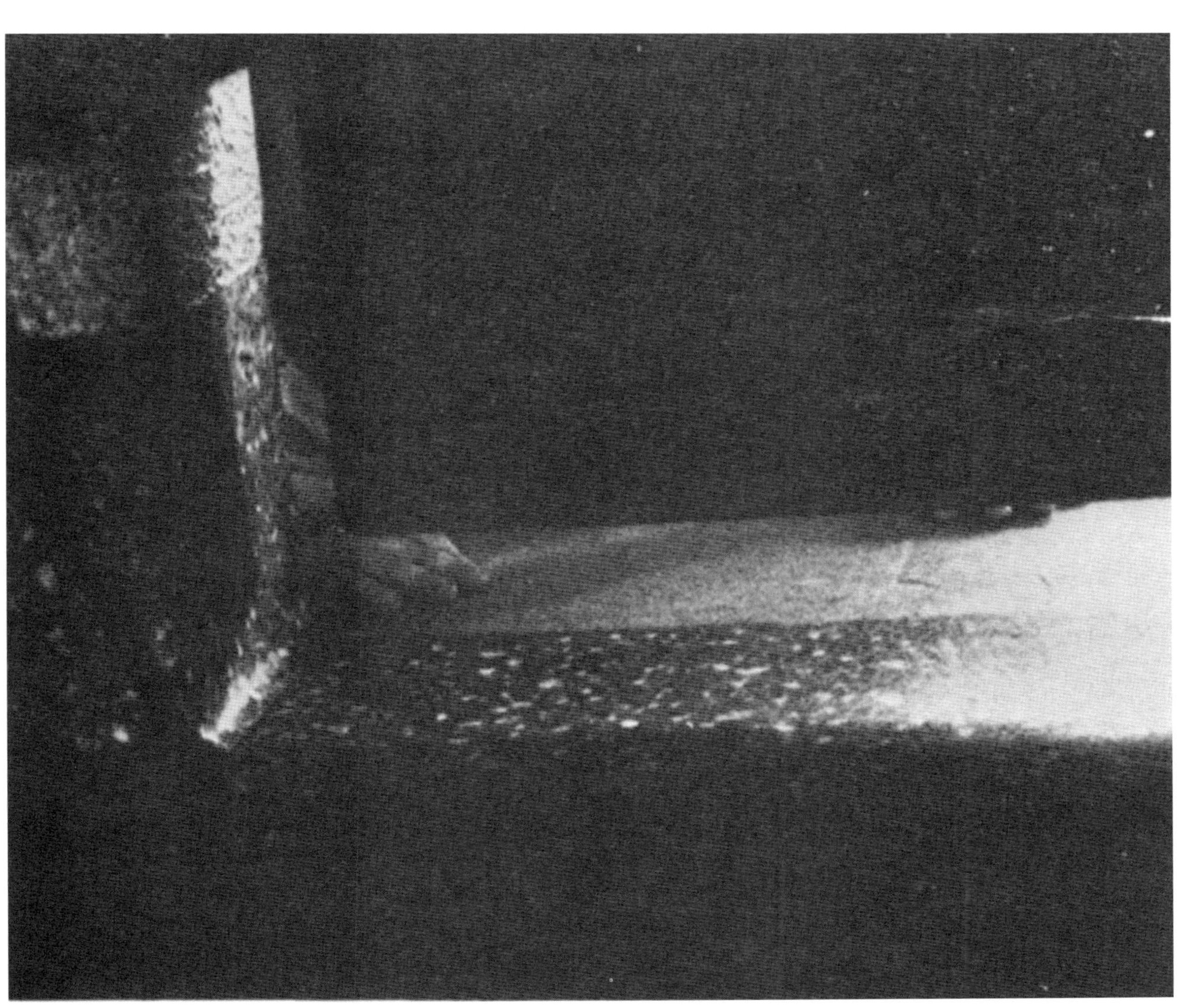

"It is not good that man should be alone."

Genesis II, 18

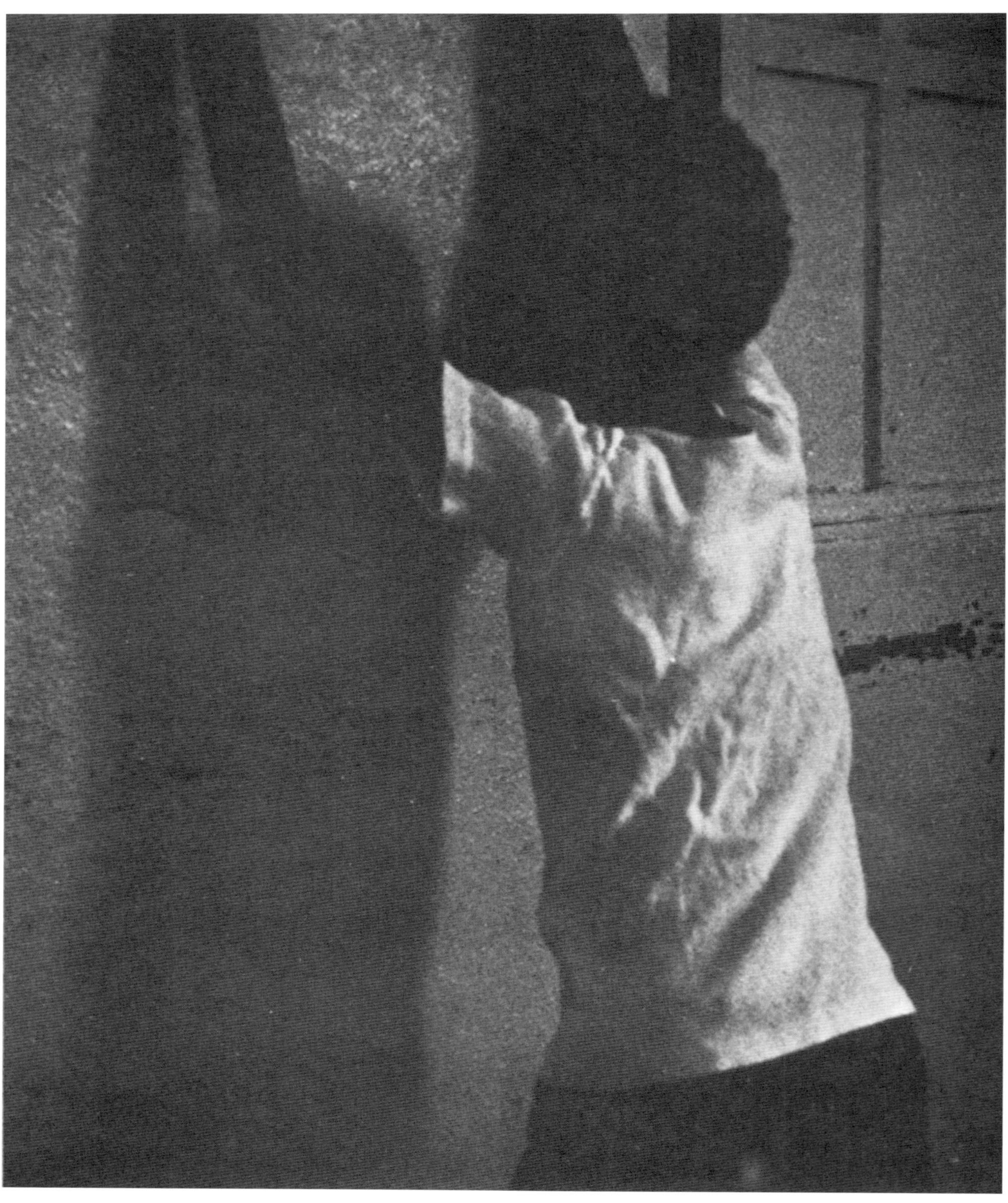

"Every one in the world is Christ and they are all
crucified."

Sherwood Anderson

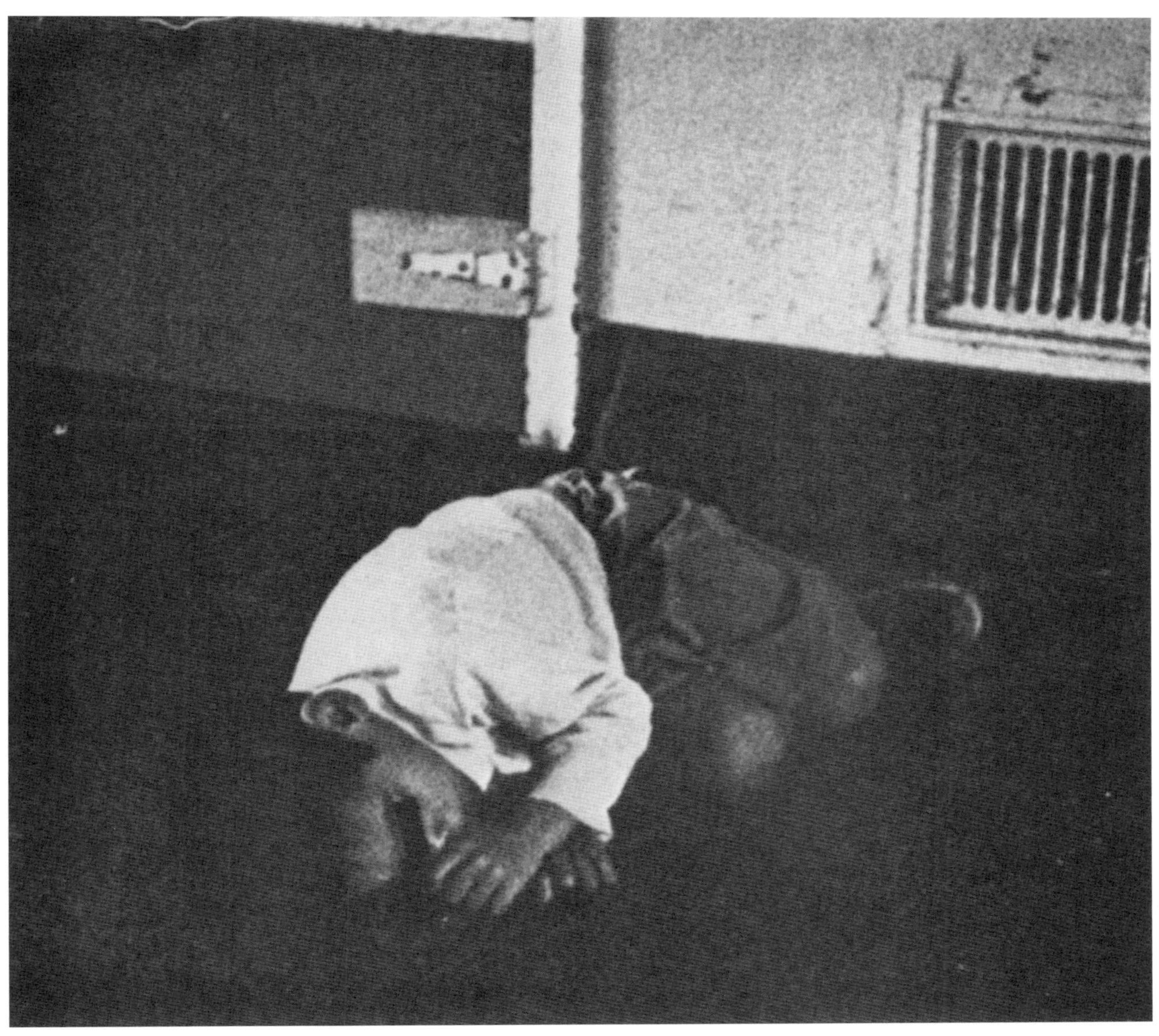

"Friday's child is full of woe."

Anonymous

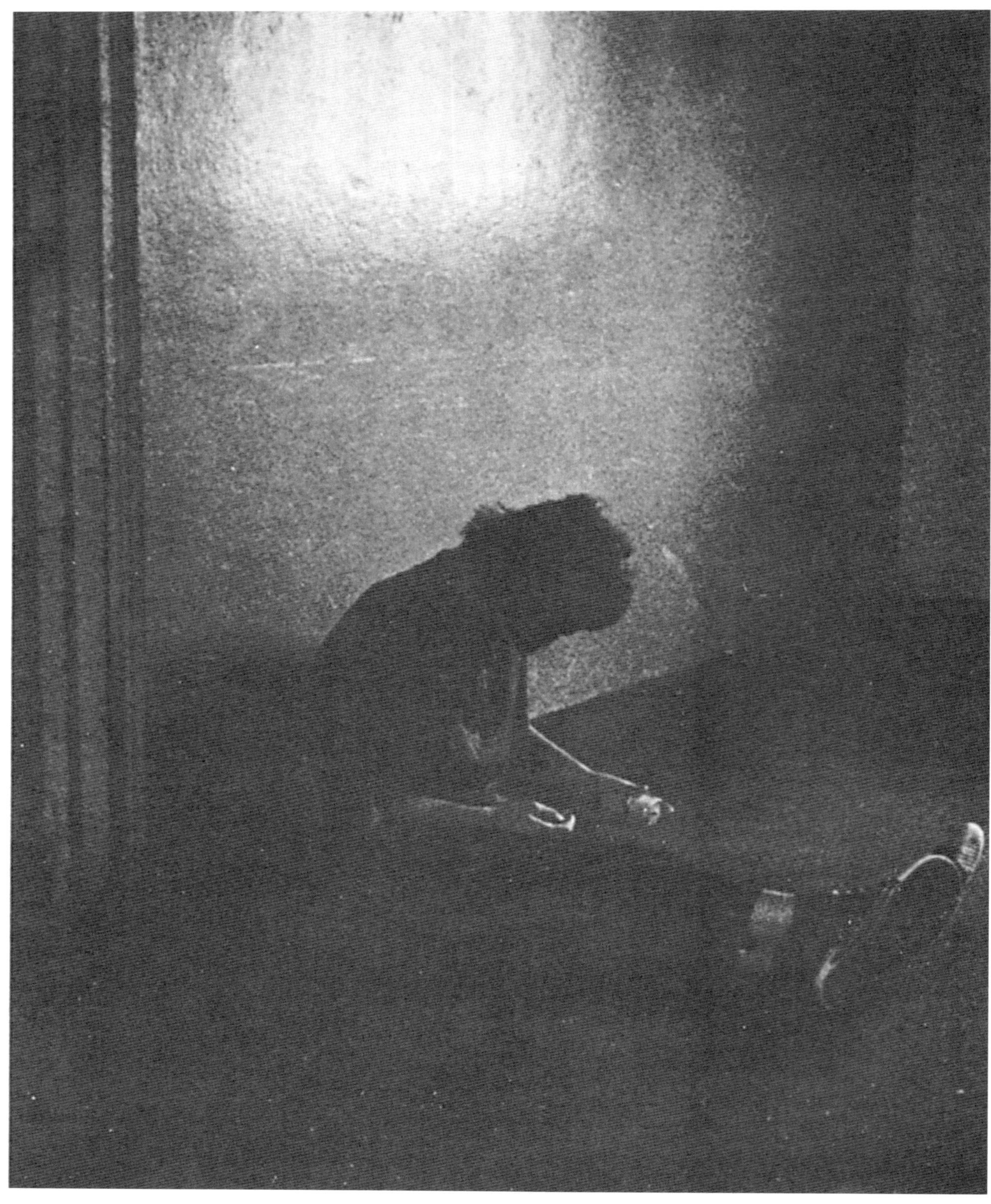

We are wrestling with our own retardation to cope, ultimately, with the retardation of others.

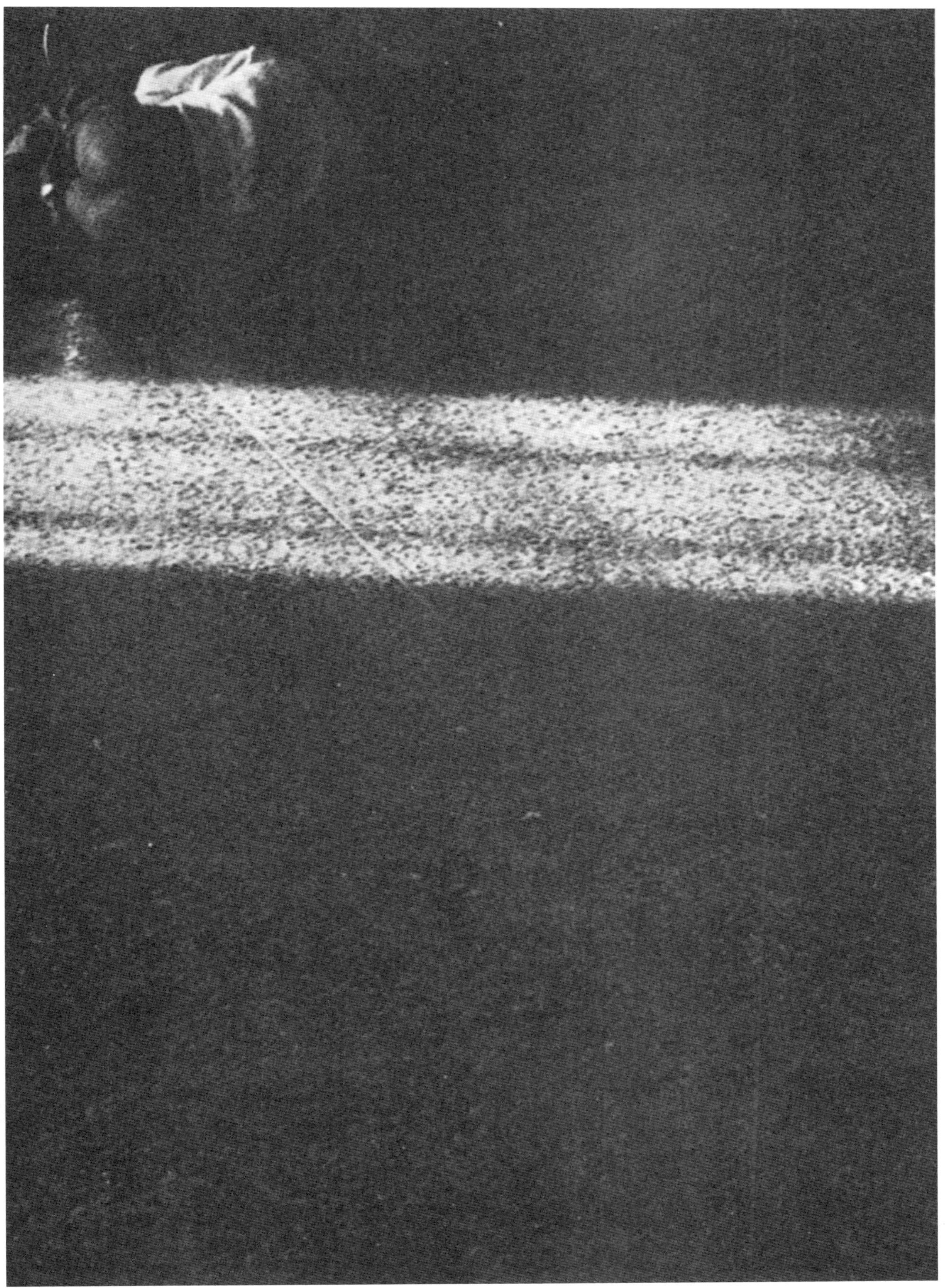

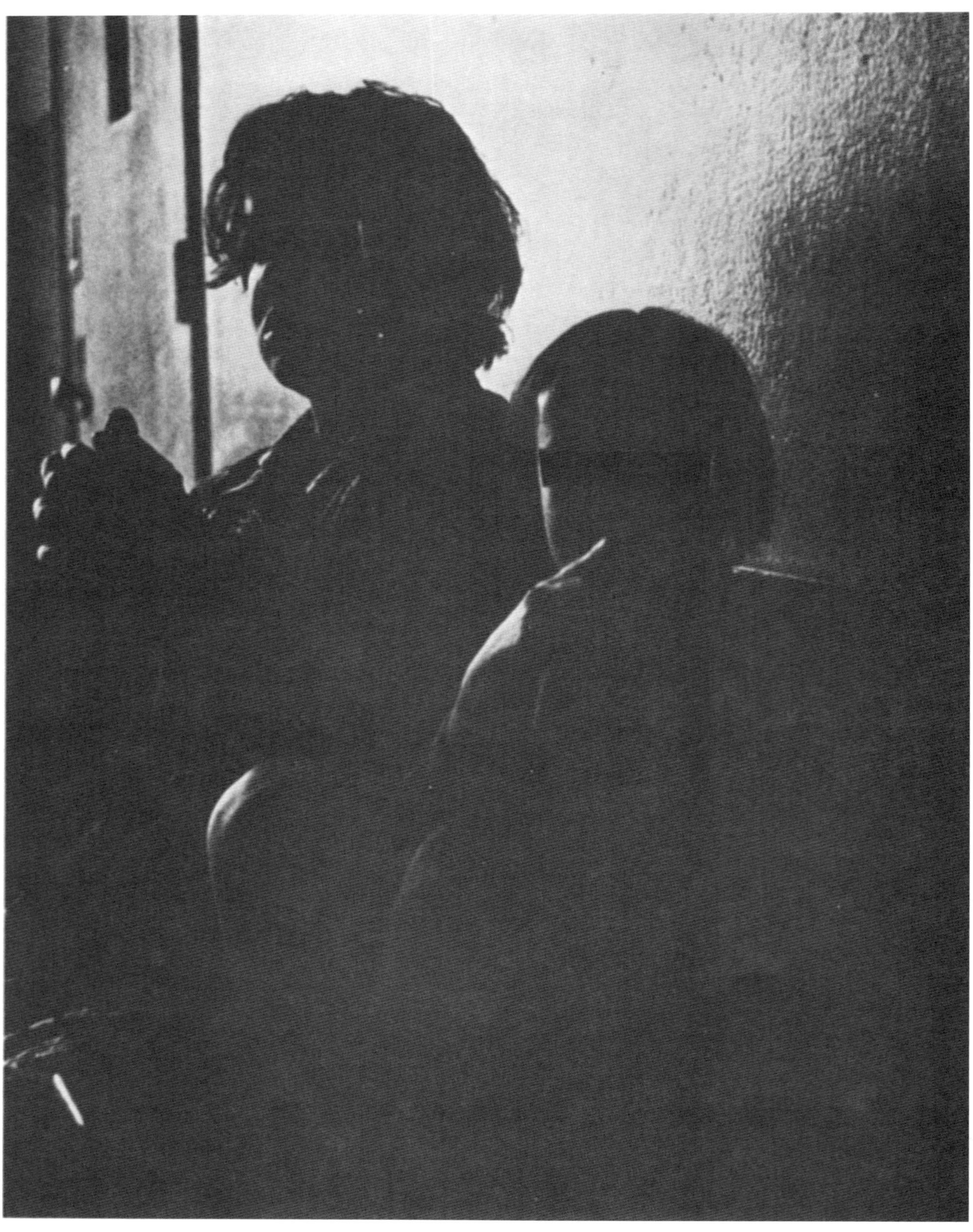

"Now we see through a glass, darkly."

1 Corinthians XIII, 12

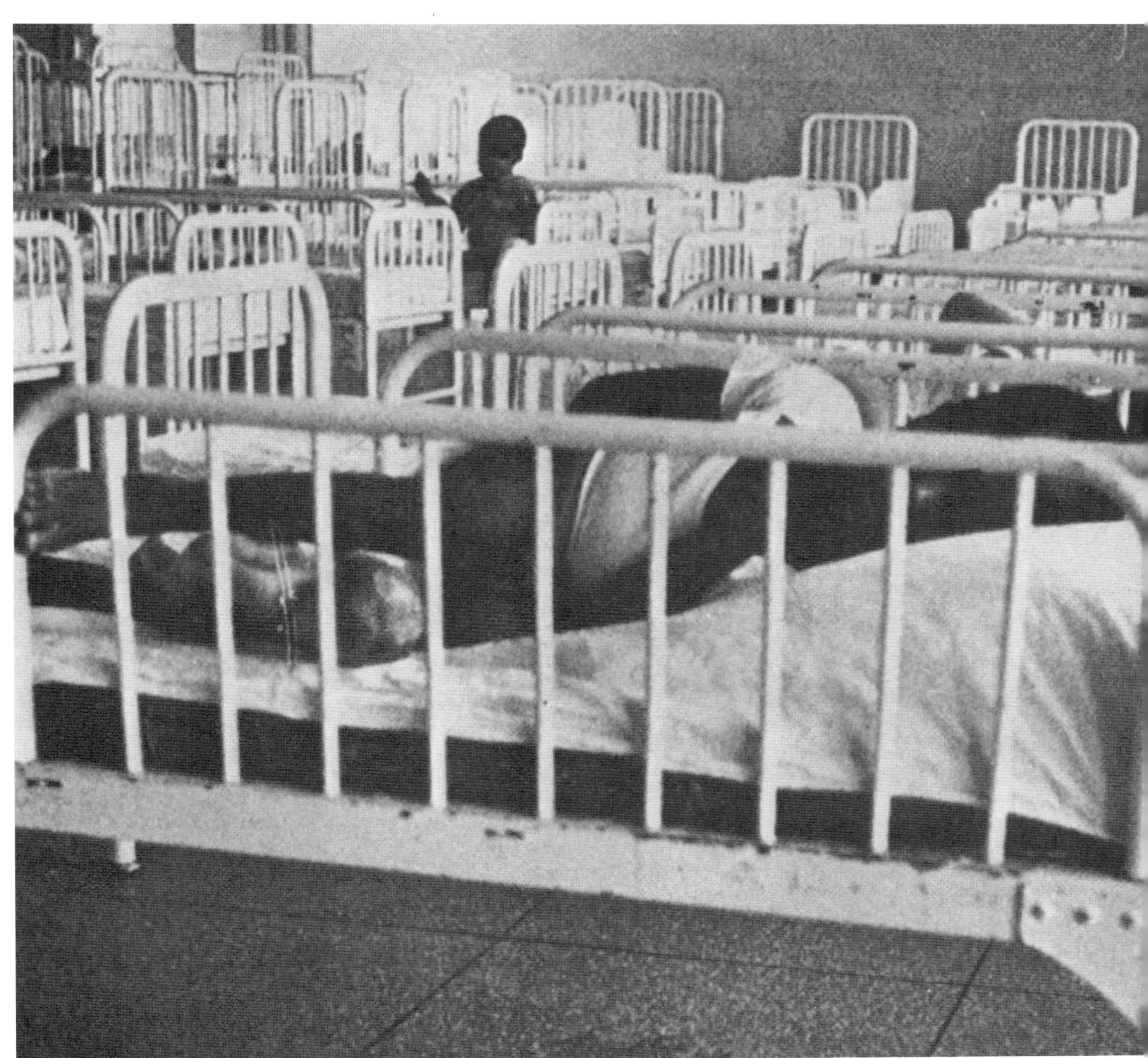

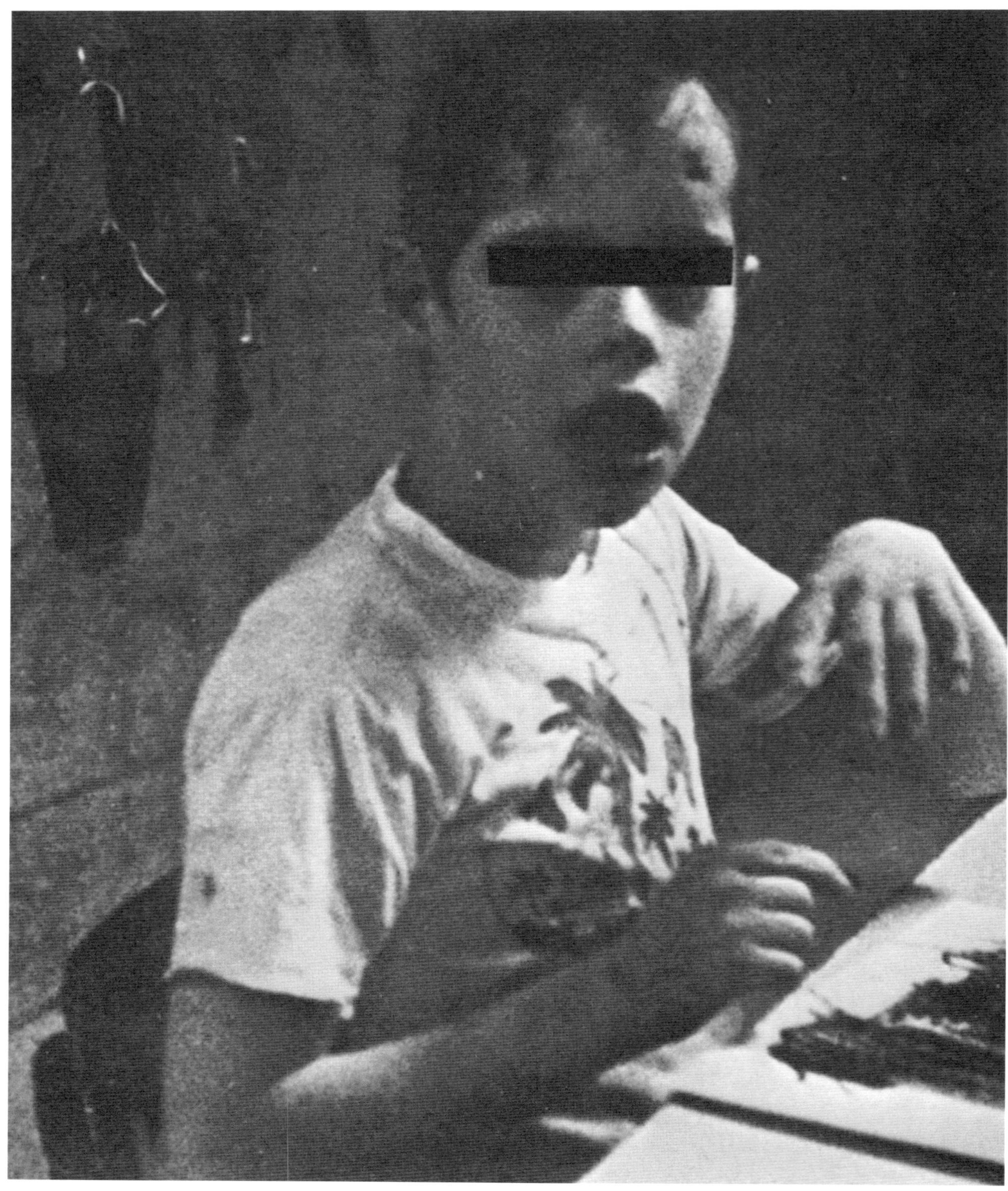

"The academic scene is now strewn with the hopes of deadened classes wherein competent teachers are stifled by children of such heterogeneity that survival becomes the major goal rather than progress. The same can be said for well-selected classes managed by poorly prepared and poorly supervised teachers. By upgrading these three areas, we can make our major contribution toward making special education something constructively special."

Herbert Goldstein

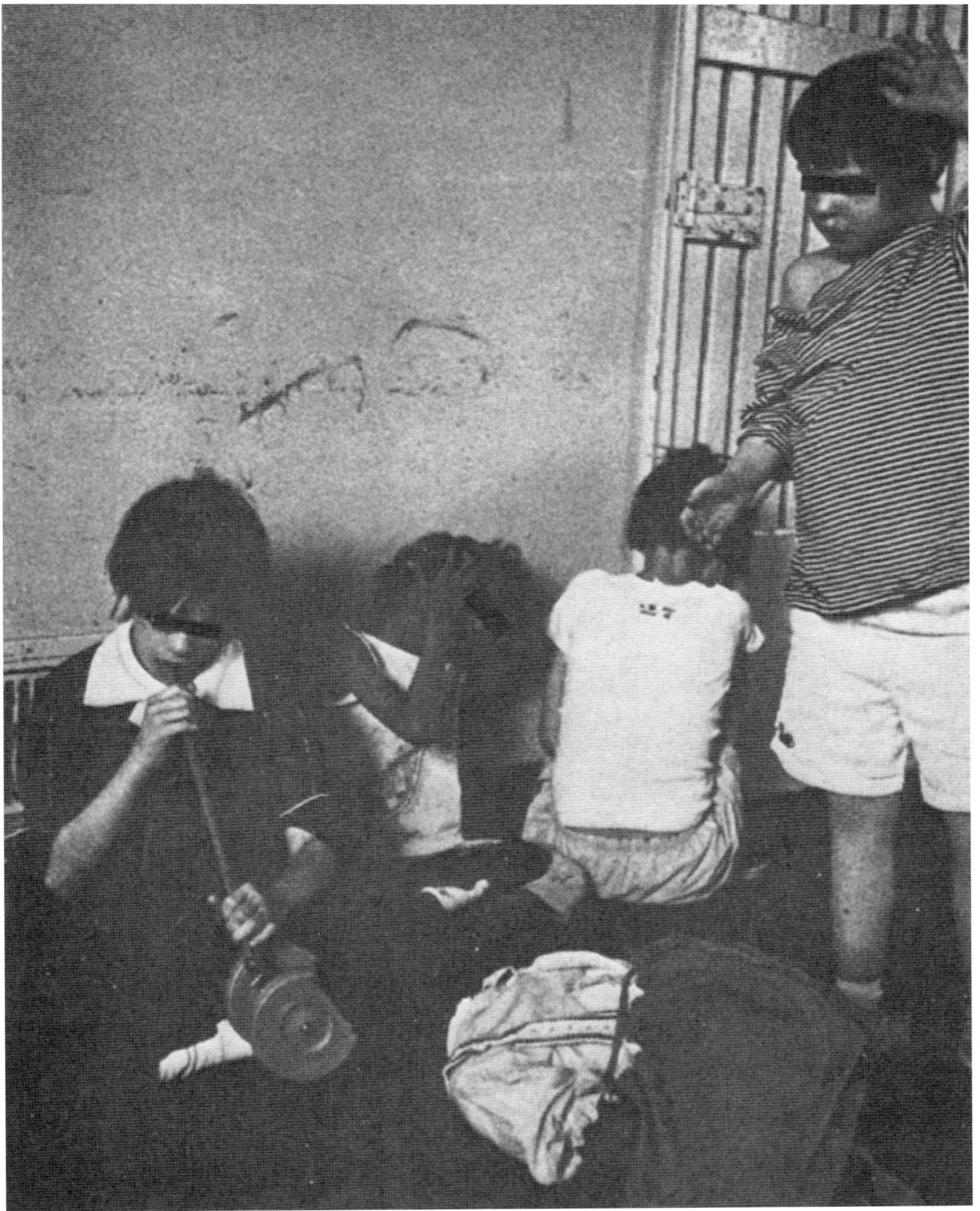

"There are only two things wrong with most special education for the mentally handicapped; it isn't special, and it isn't education."

Alice Metzner

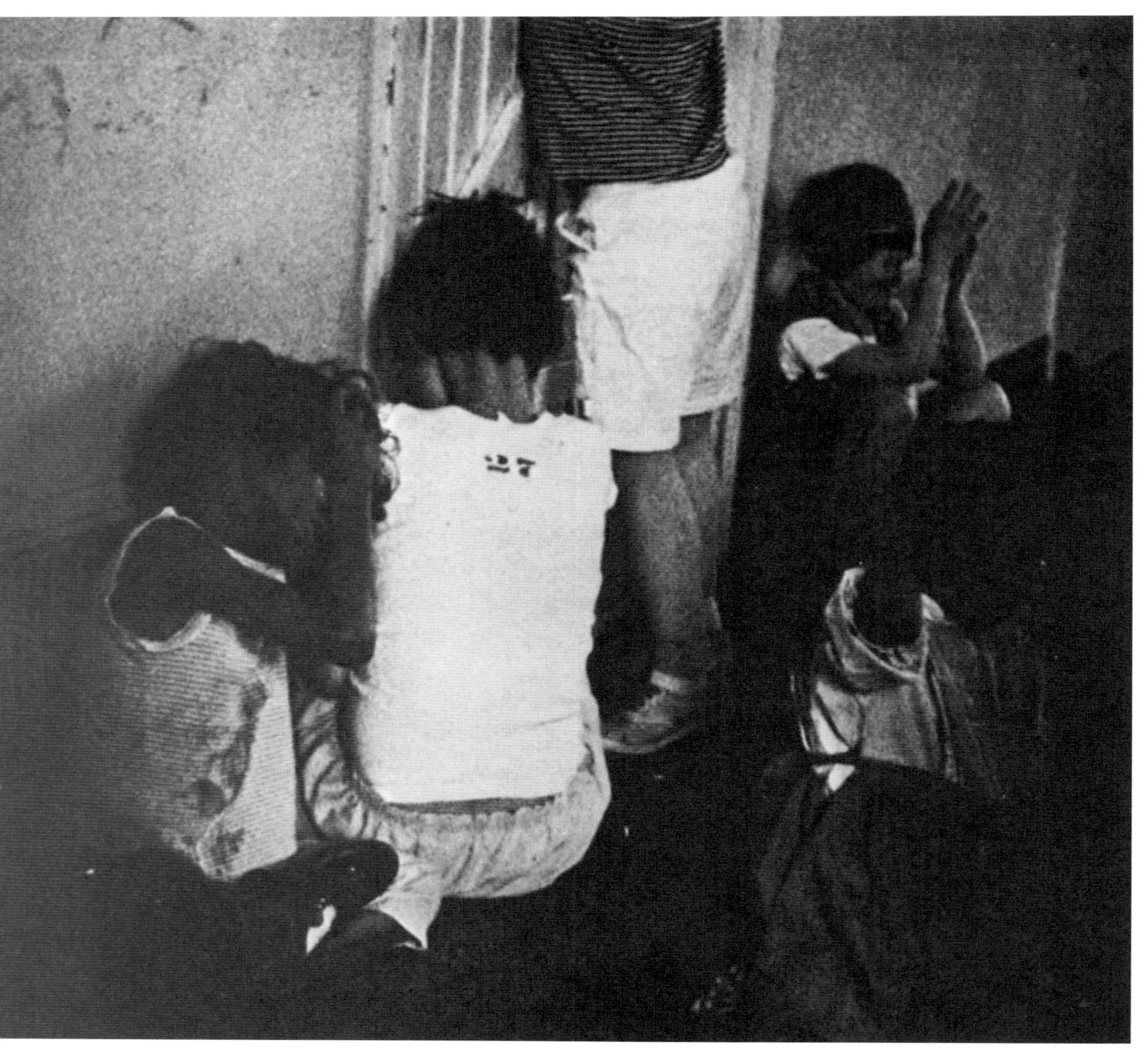

"...the offspring of the inferior, or of the better when they chance to be deformed, will be put away in some mysterious, unknown place..."

Plato

# "The wretched souls…"

"The wretched souls of those who lived
Without all praise or blame."

Dante

The living quarters for older men and women were, for the most part, gloomy and sterile. There were rows and rows of benches on which sat countless human beings, in silent rooms, waiting for dinner call or bedtime. We saw resident after resident in "institutional garb." Sometimes, the women wore shrouds—inside out.

We heard a good deal of laughter but saw little cheer. There were few things to be cheerful about. A great many of the men and women looked depressed and acted depressed. Even the television sets, in several of the day rooms, appeared to be co-conspirators in a crusade for gloom. These sets were not in working order. Sadly, the residents continued to sit on their benches, in neat rows, looking at the blank tubes.

We observed adult residents during recreation, playing "ring-around the-rosy." Others, in the vocational training center, were playing "jacks." These were not always severely retarded patients. However, we got the feeling very quickly that this is the way they were being forced to behave.

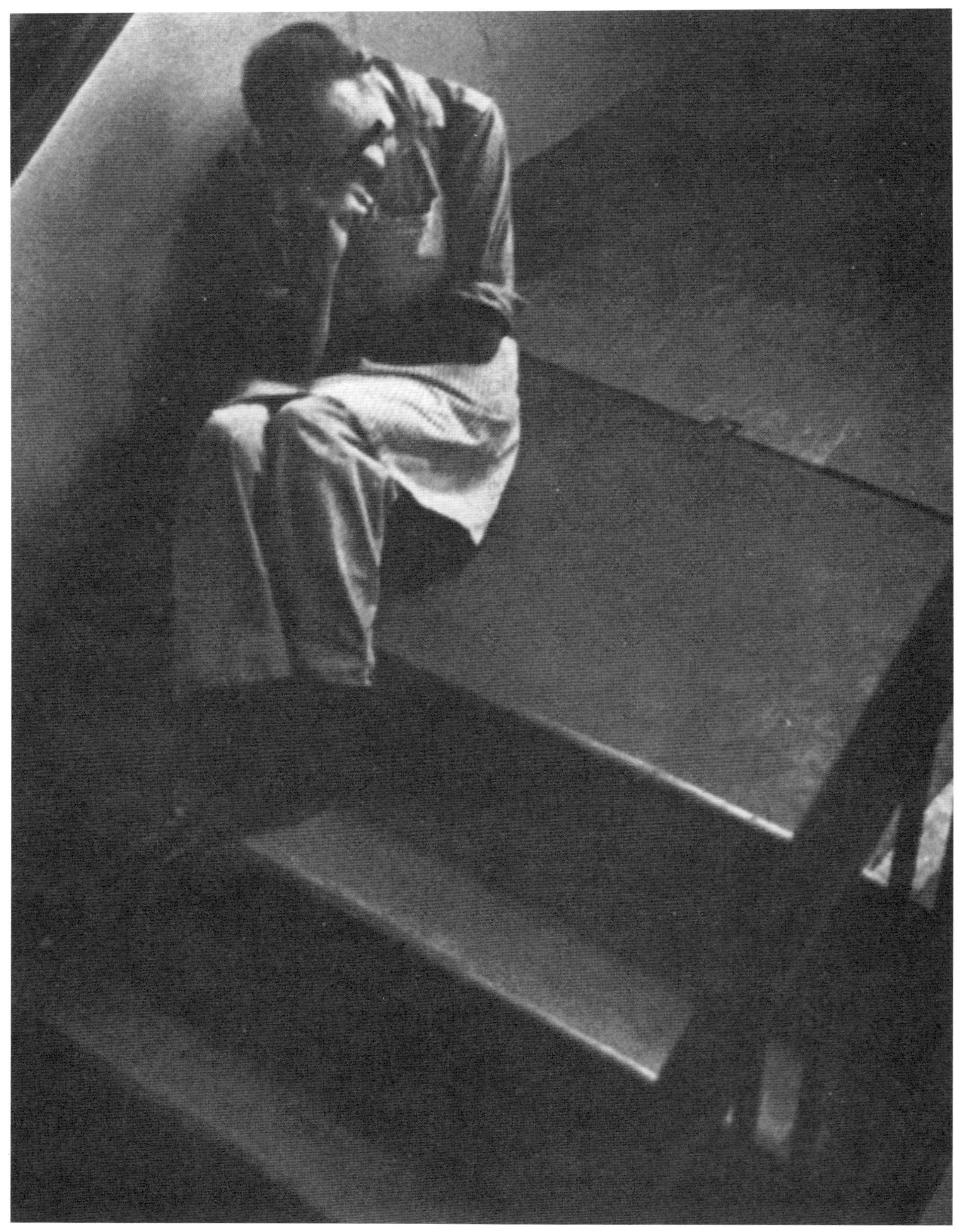

"My friends forsake me like a memory lost."

John Clare

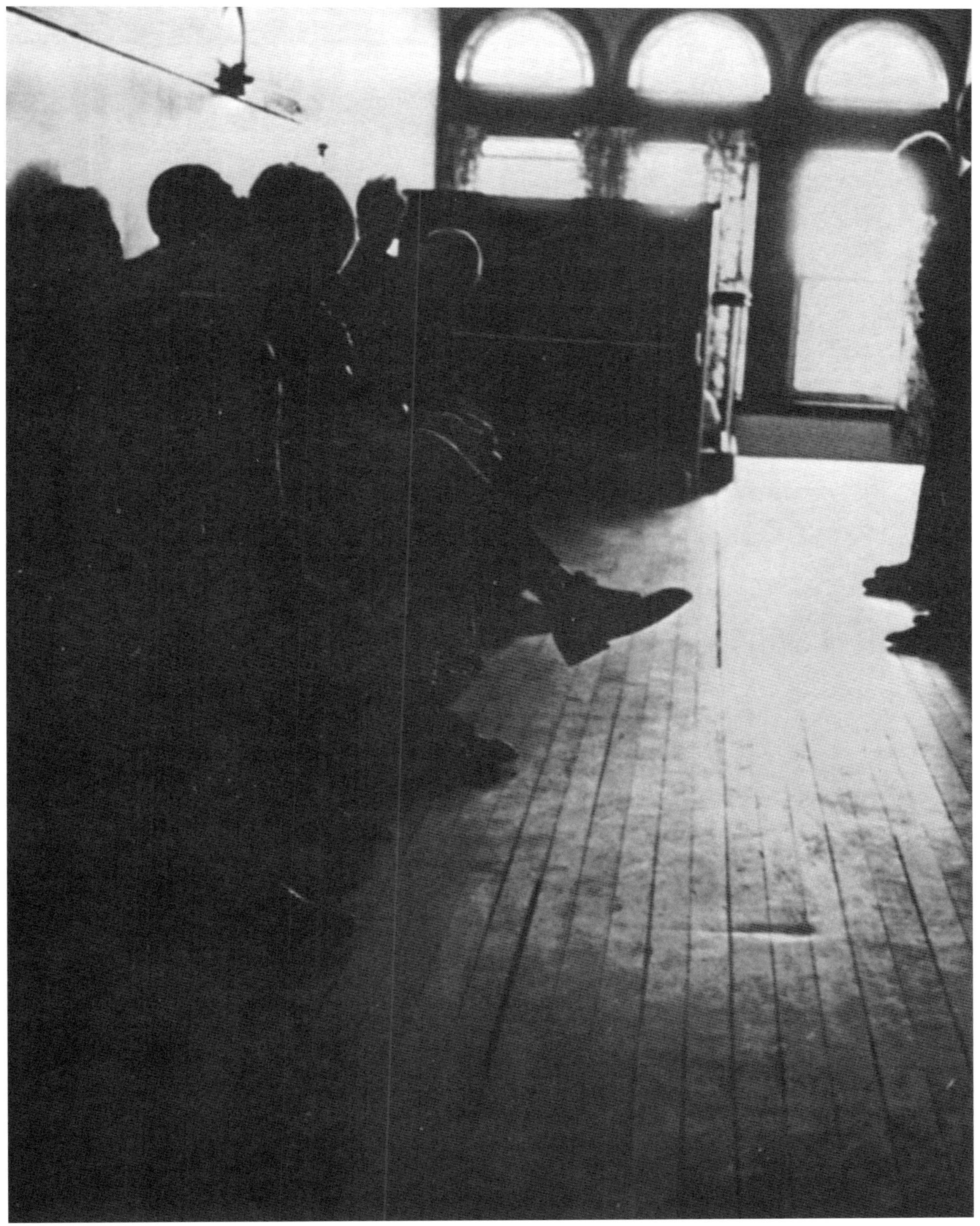

"…in an institution there is always tomorrow so that he who starts out a student ends up, by default, an inmate."

Richard H. Hungerford

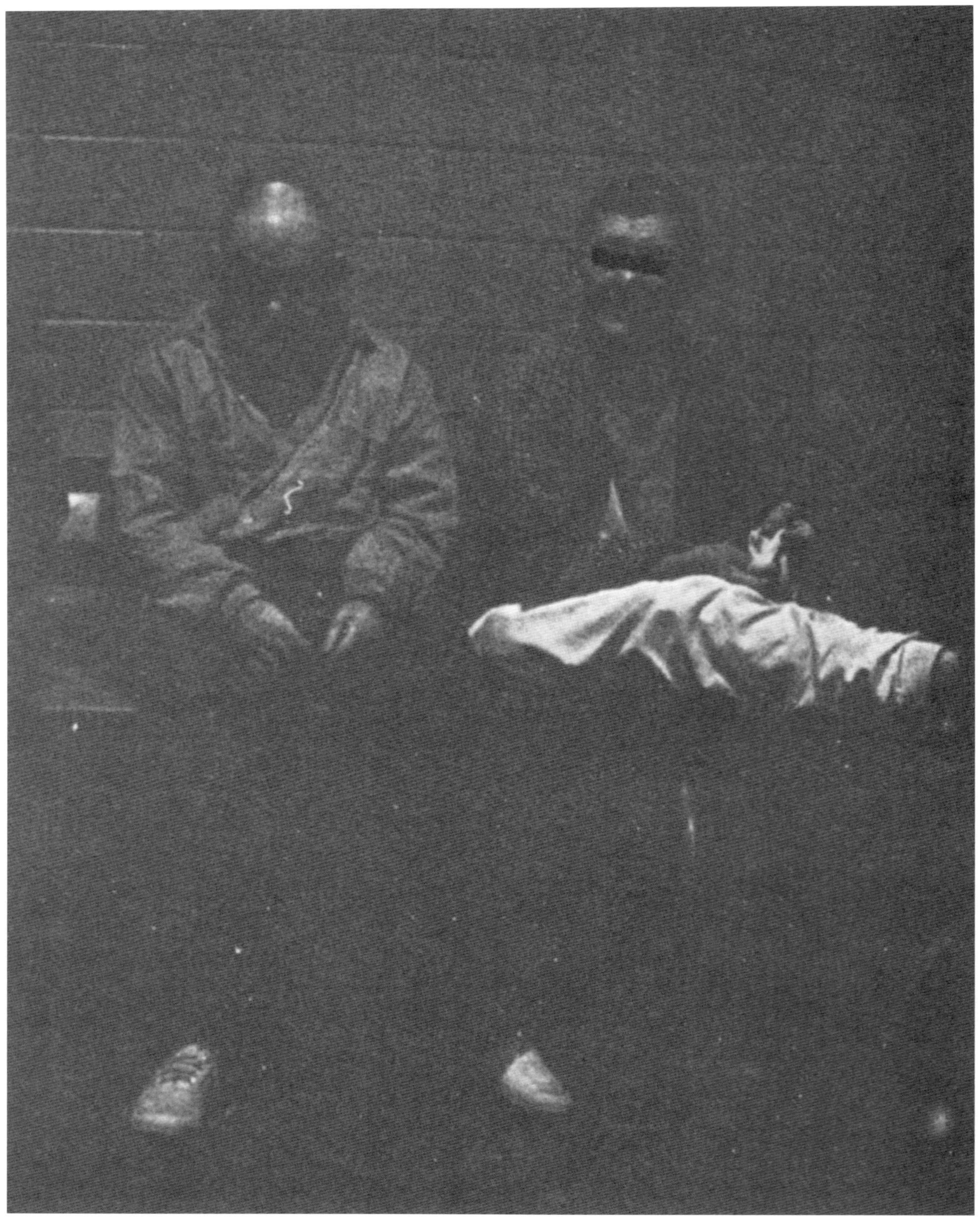

"Where'er men go, in heaven, or earth, or hell
They find themselves, and that is all they find."

Samuel Valentine Cole

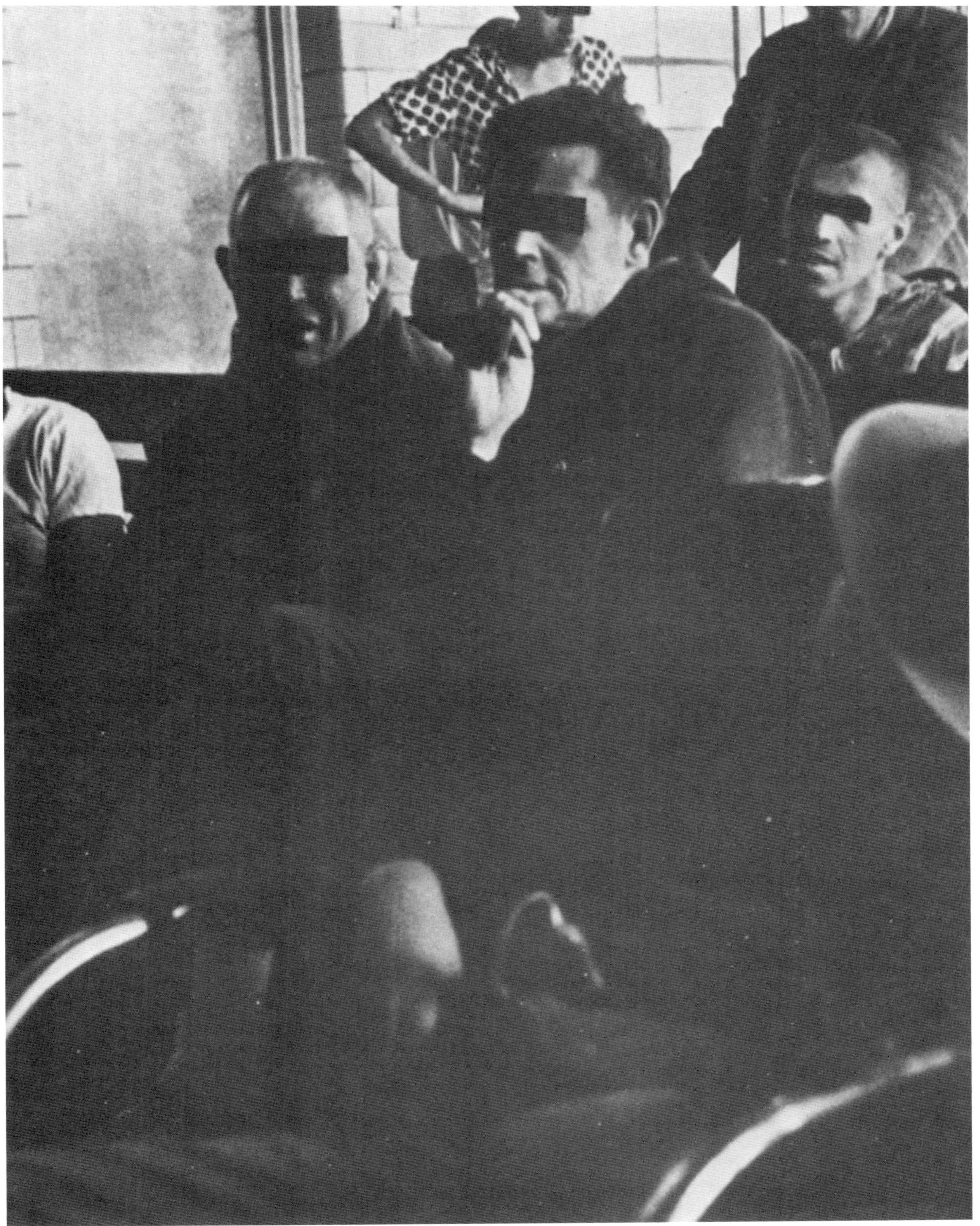

"Man is a pliable animal, a being who gets accustomed to everything!"

Fyodor Dostoyevsky

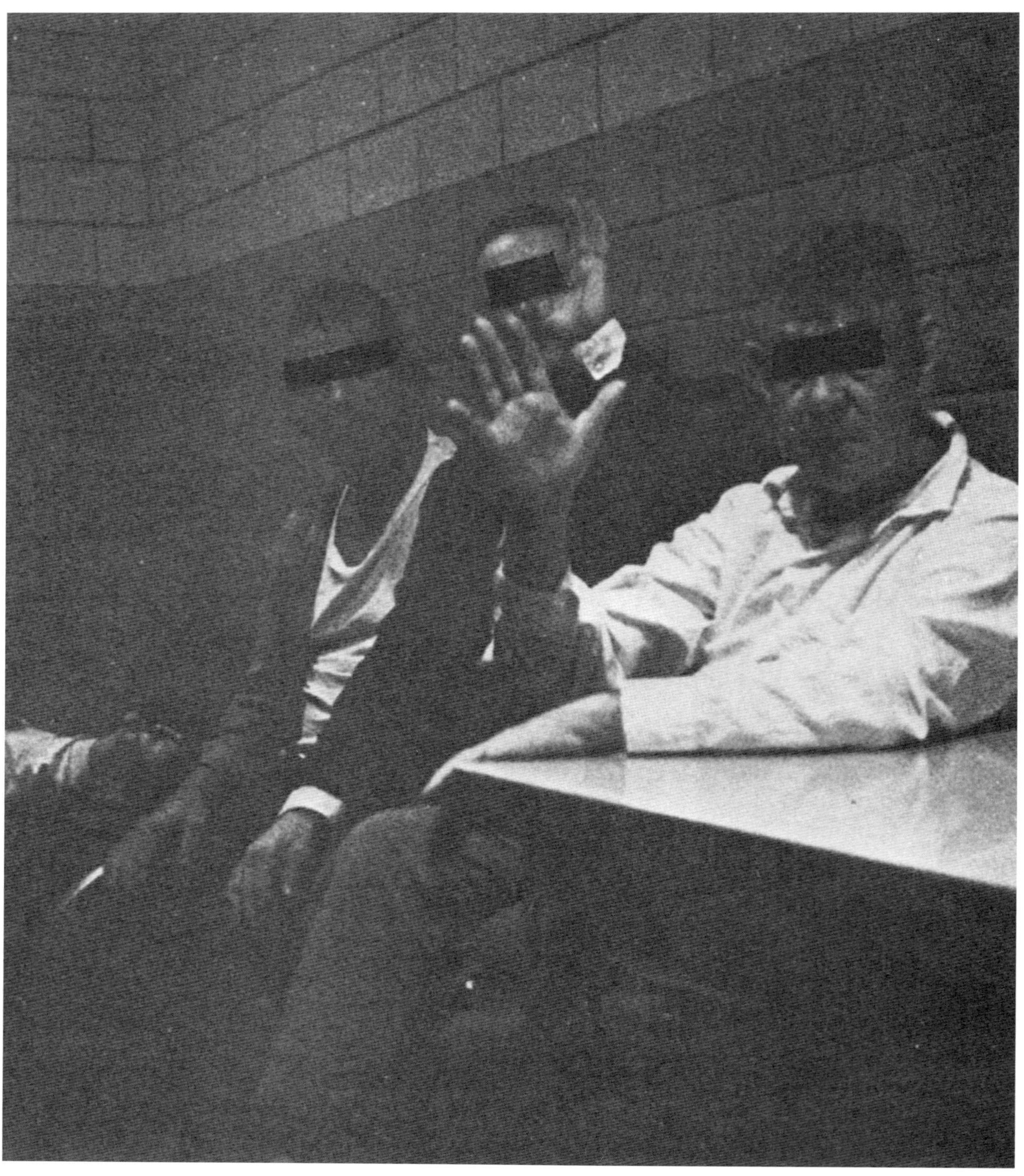

"'We lock these unfortunate creatures in lunatic cells, as if they were criminals,' exclaimed Reil in 1803, 'We keep them in chains in forlorn jails, near the roosts of owls in hidden recesses above the gates of towns, or in the damp cellars of reformatories where no sympathetic human being can ever bestow them a friendly glance, and we let them rot in their own filth. There fetters scrape the flesh from their bones, and their wan, hollow faces search for the grave that their wailing and our ignominy conceals from them.'"

Emil Kraepelin

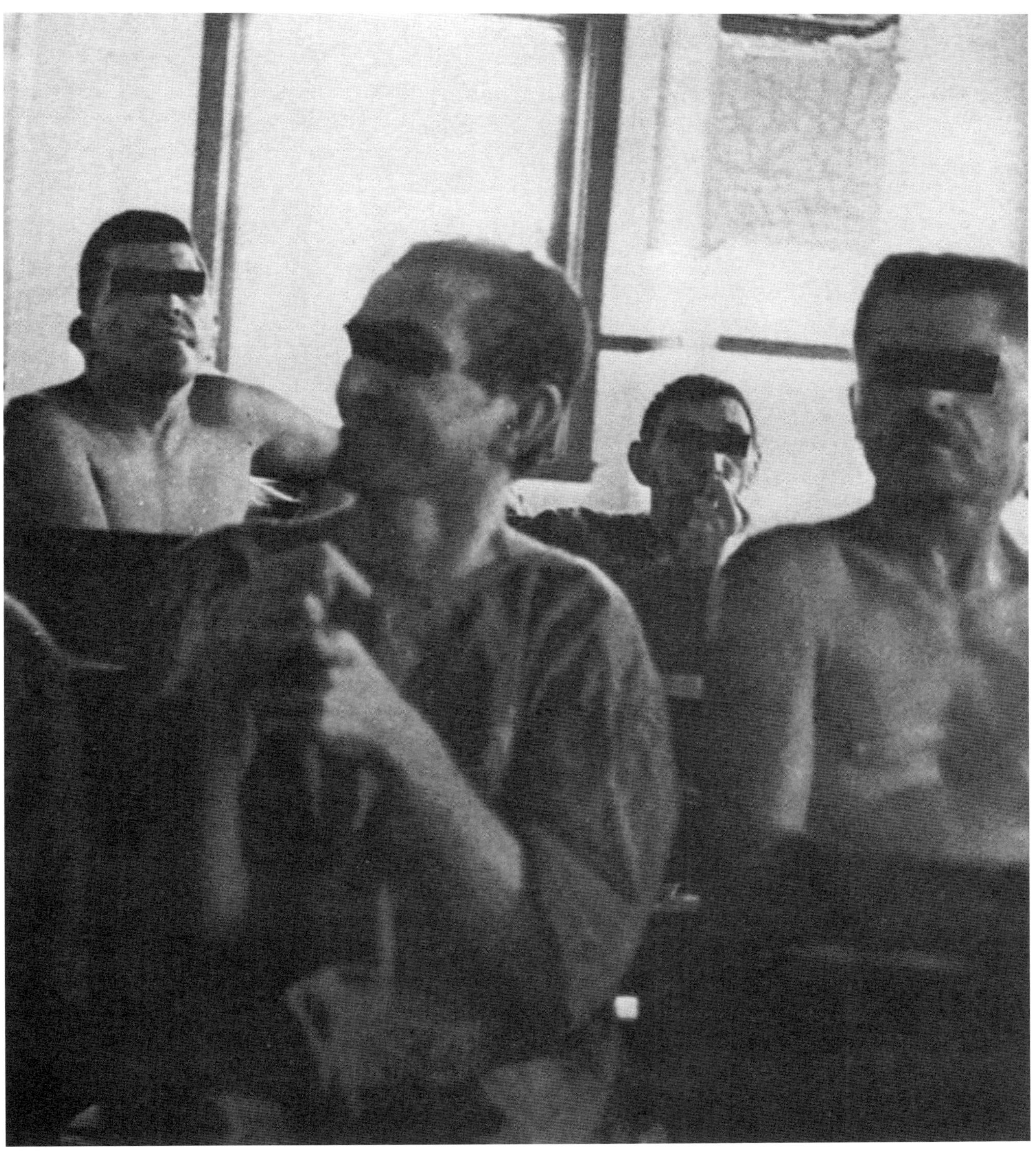

"Our troubles emanate not from biological idiots but from social ones; and social idiots are produced by society, not by genes. It is therefore the social, not biological, therapy that is indicated."

Ashley Montagu

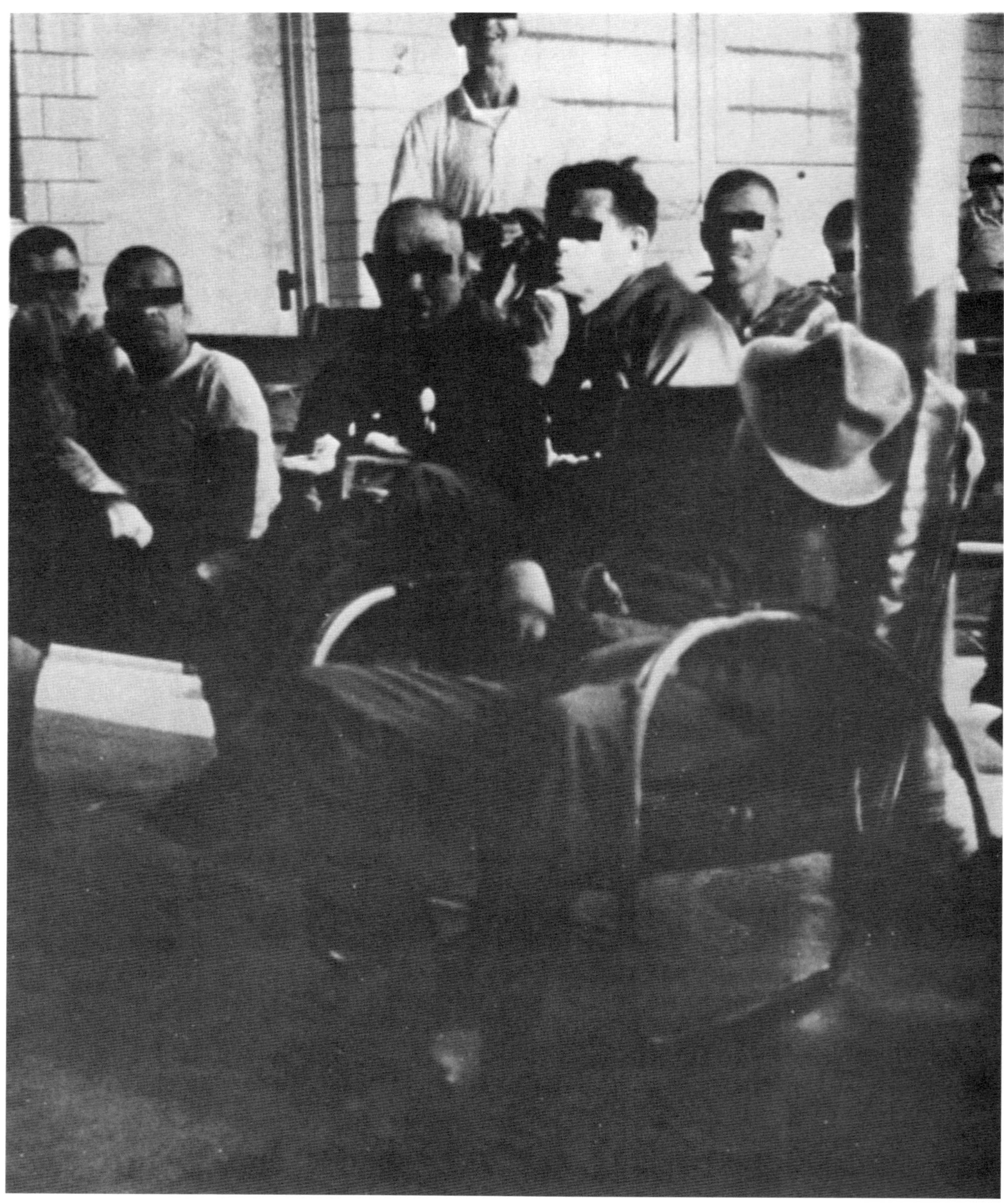

"No man is an Island, intire of inselfe; every man is
a peece of the Continent, a part of the maine..."

John Donne

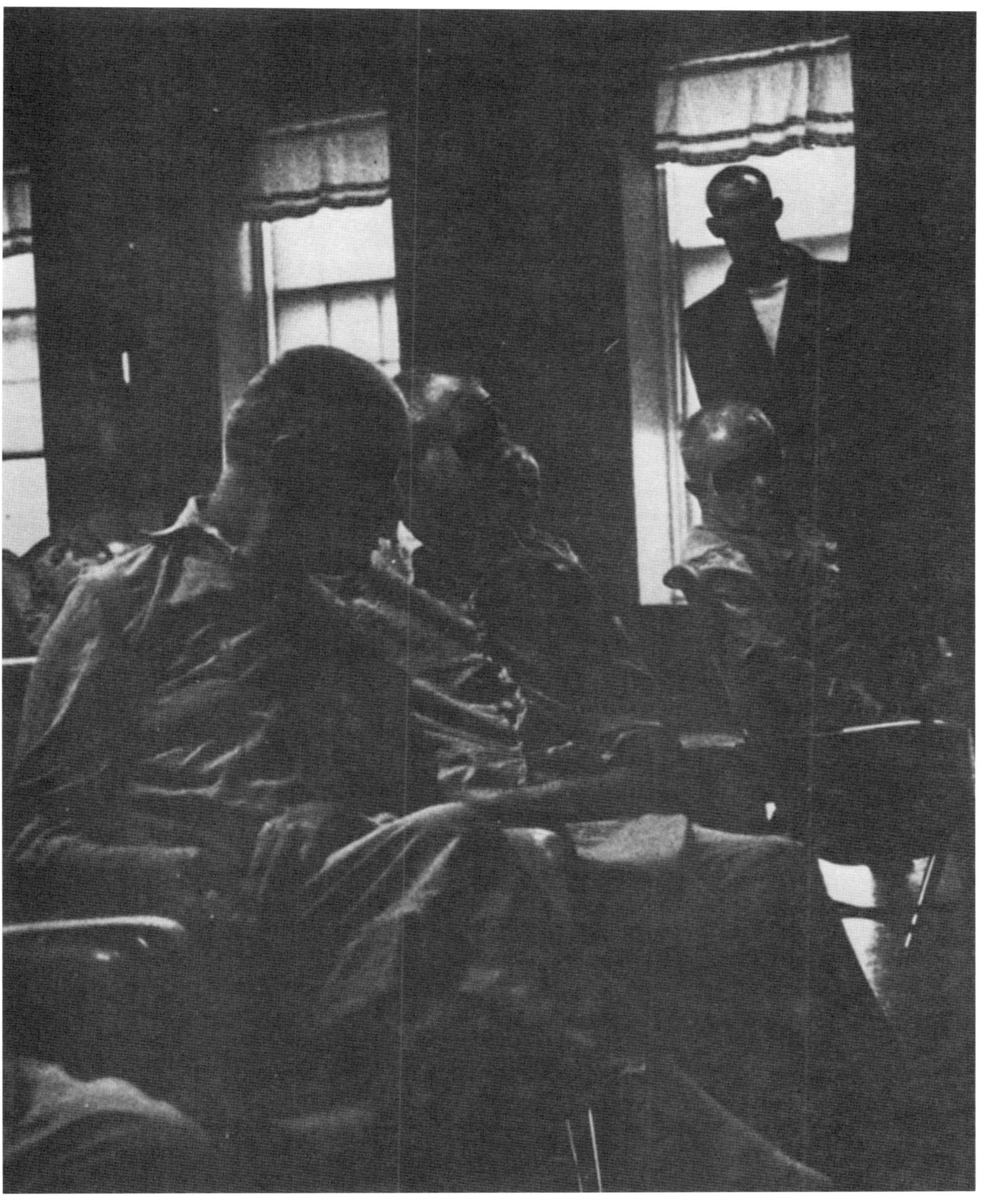

"Until you have become really, in actual fact, a brother to every one, brotherhood will not come to pass."

Fyodor Dostoyevsky

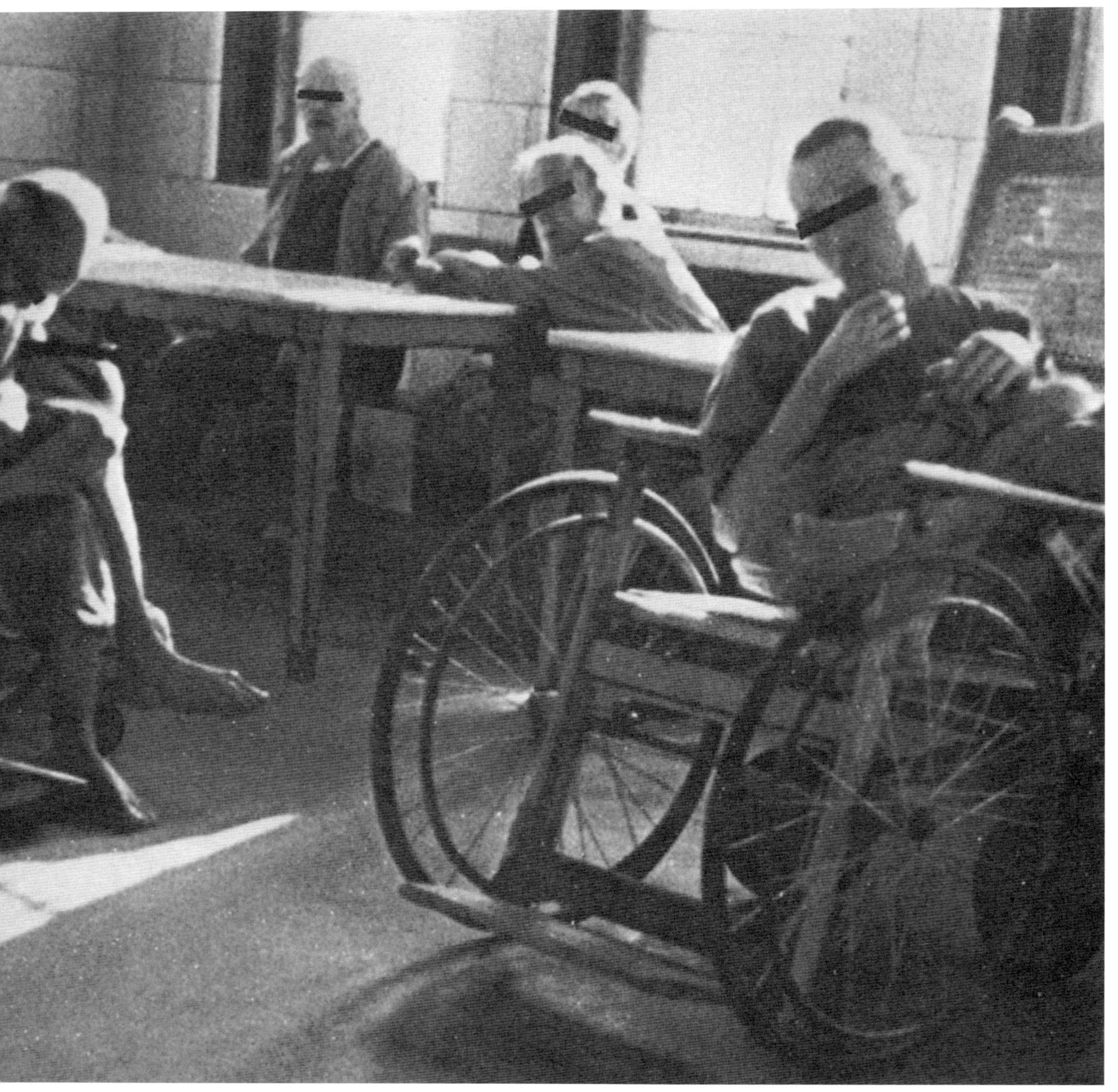

"One handicap tends to beget another."

Albert T. Murphy

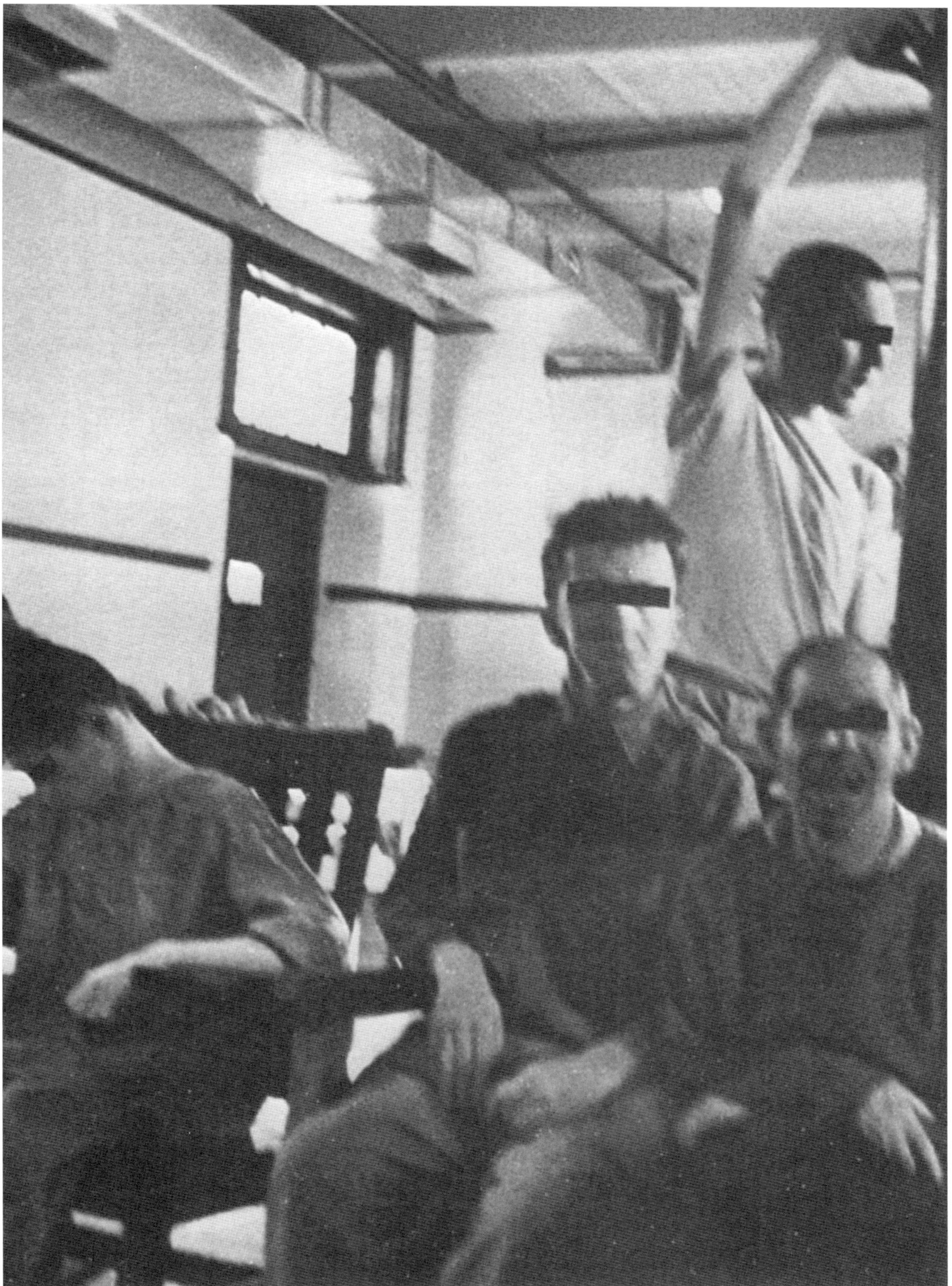

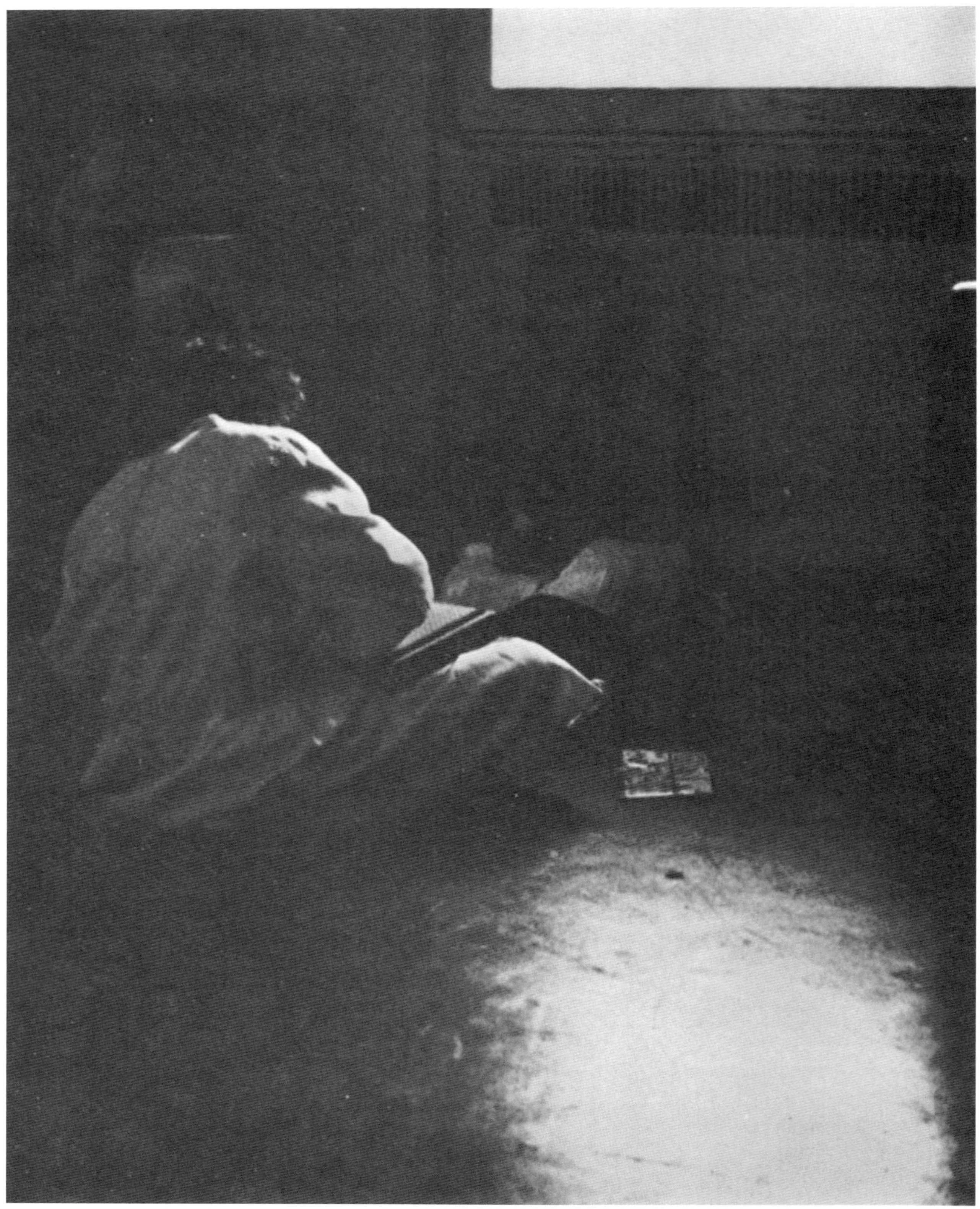

"God hath chosen the foolish things of the world to confound the wise; and God hath chosen the weak things of the world to confound the things which are mighty."

1 Corinthians I, 27

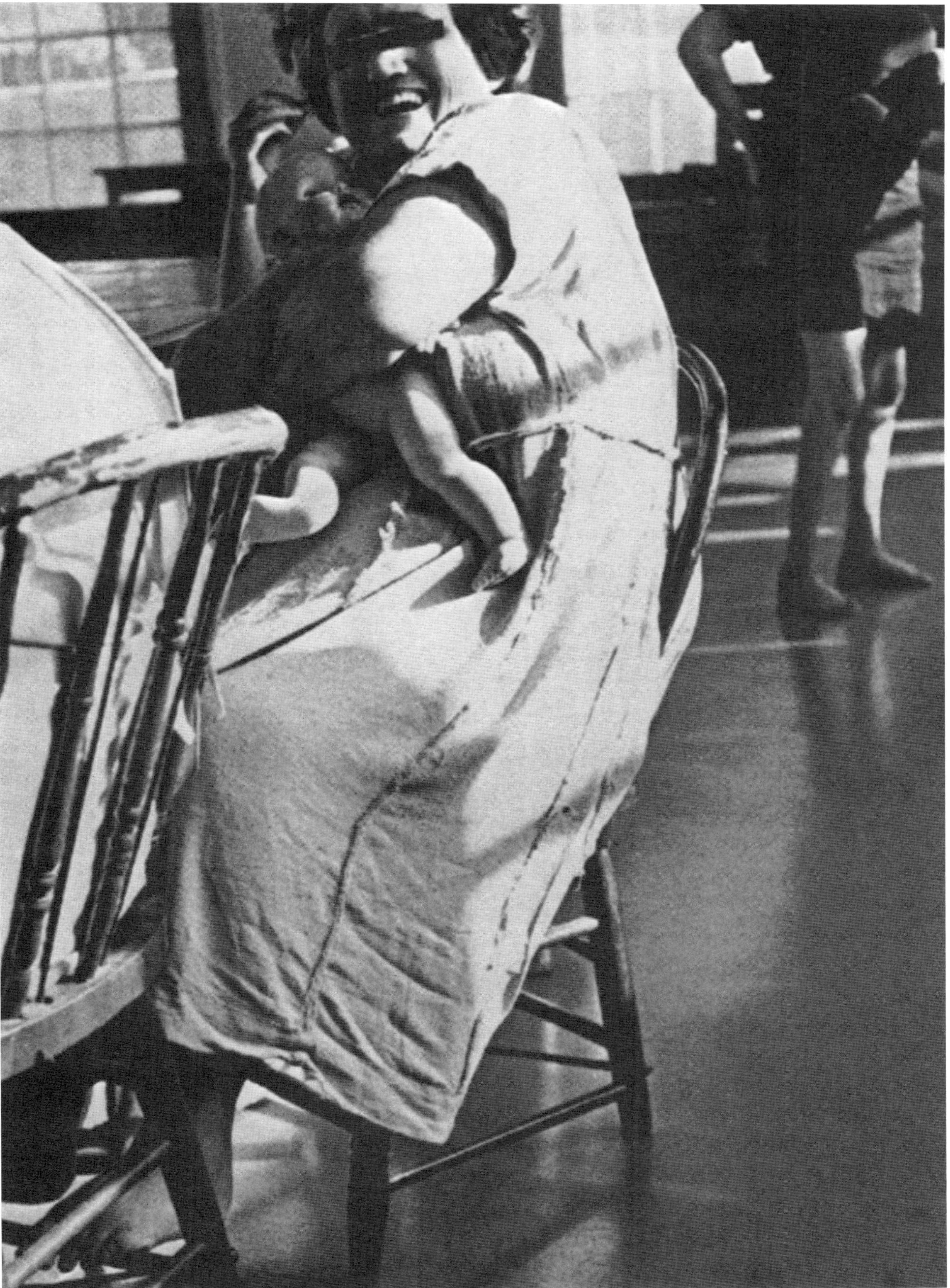

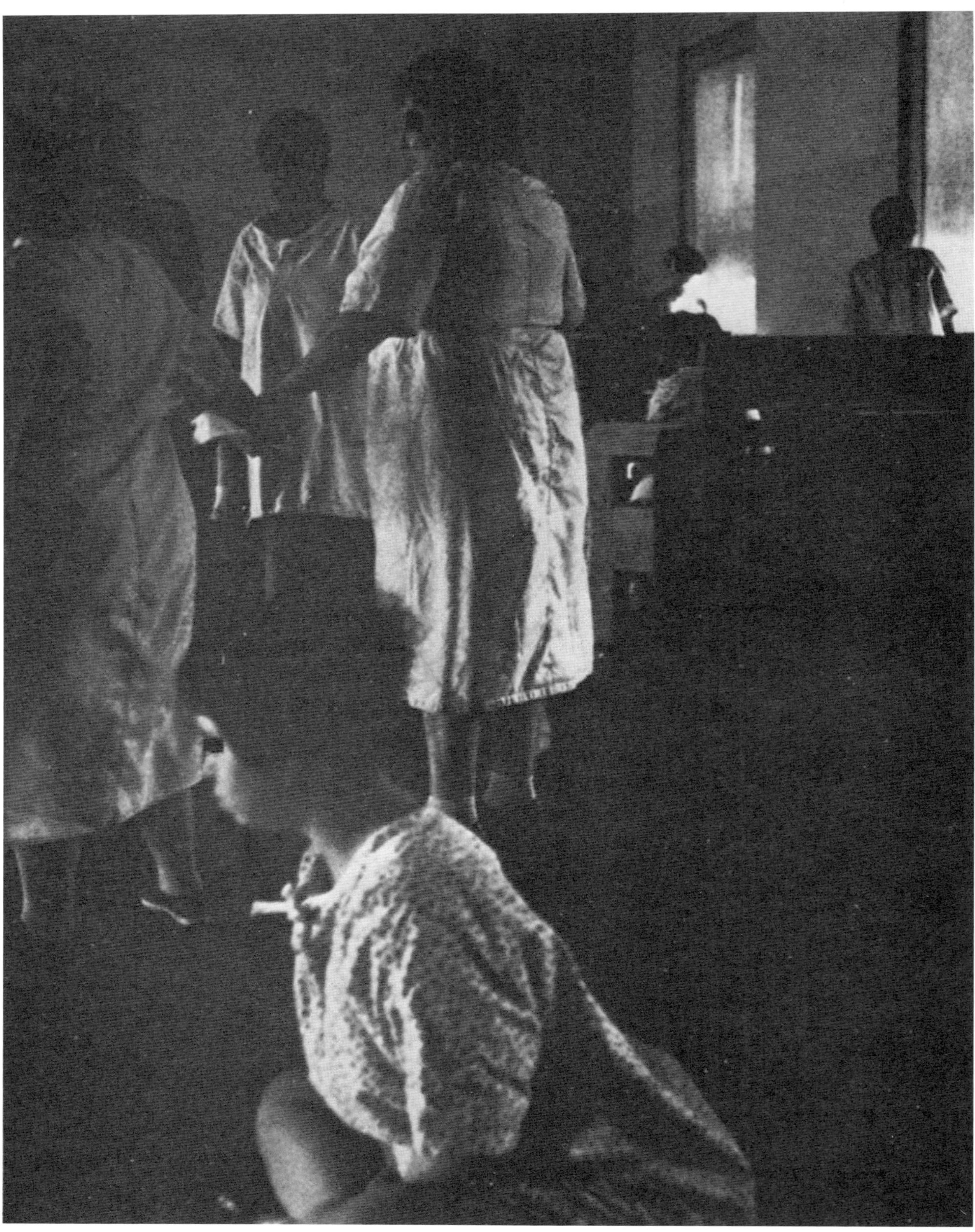

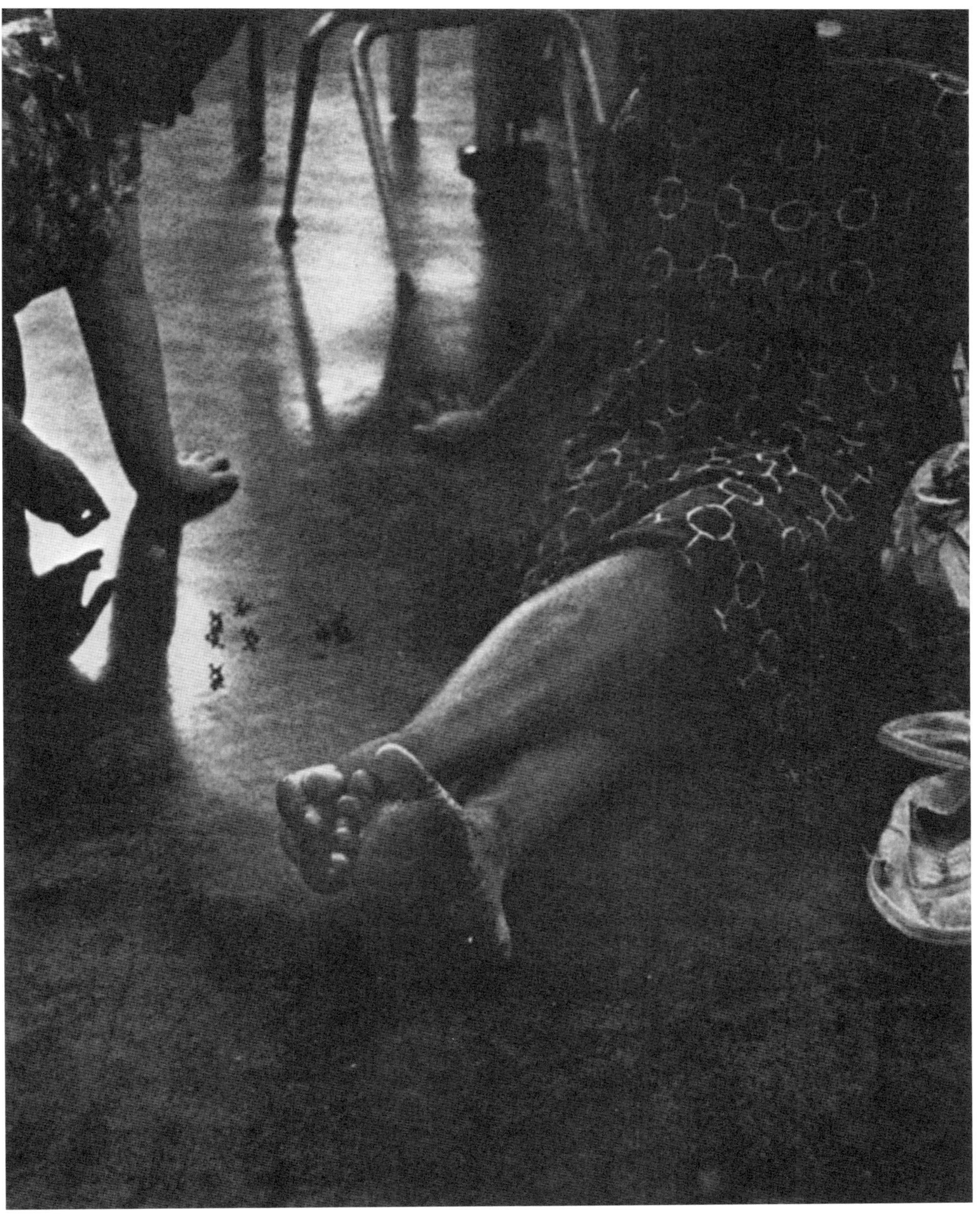

"Time buries the mistakes of many school programs."

Richard H. Hungerford

# "In bed we laugh…"

"In bed we laugh, in bed we cry;
And, born in bed, in bed we die.
The near approach a bed may show
Of human bliss to human woe."

Isaac de Benserade

Among the things we will remember are the beds and the benches. Early in the evening, sometimes as early as 5 P.M., patients are put to bed. This is to equalize the work load among the different attendant shifts. During the day, we saw many patients lying on their beds, apparently for long periods of time. This was their activity.

During these observations, we thought a great deal about the perennial cry for attendants and volunteer workers who are more sympathetic and understanding of institutionalized retarded residents. One of the things we realized was that attendants might be sympathetic, might interact more with patients, if institutional administrators made deliberate attempts to make patients cosmetically more appealing. For example, male adult residents should shave—or be shaven—more than once or twice a week. Dentures should be provided for any patient who needs them. It seems plausible to believe that it is much more possible to make residents more attractive and, therefore, more interesting to attendants than it is to attempt to convince attendants that they should enjoy the spectacle of unwashed, unkempt, odoriferous, toothless old men and women.

Lastly, we viewed old women and very young girls in the same dormitories and old men and young boys as comrades in the day room. In the "normal" world, there is something appealing—even touching—about such friendships. In an institution residents would benefit by companionship from patients their own age.

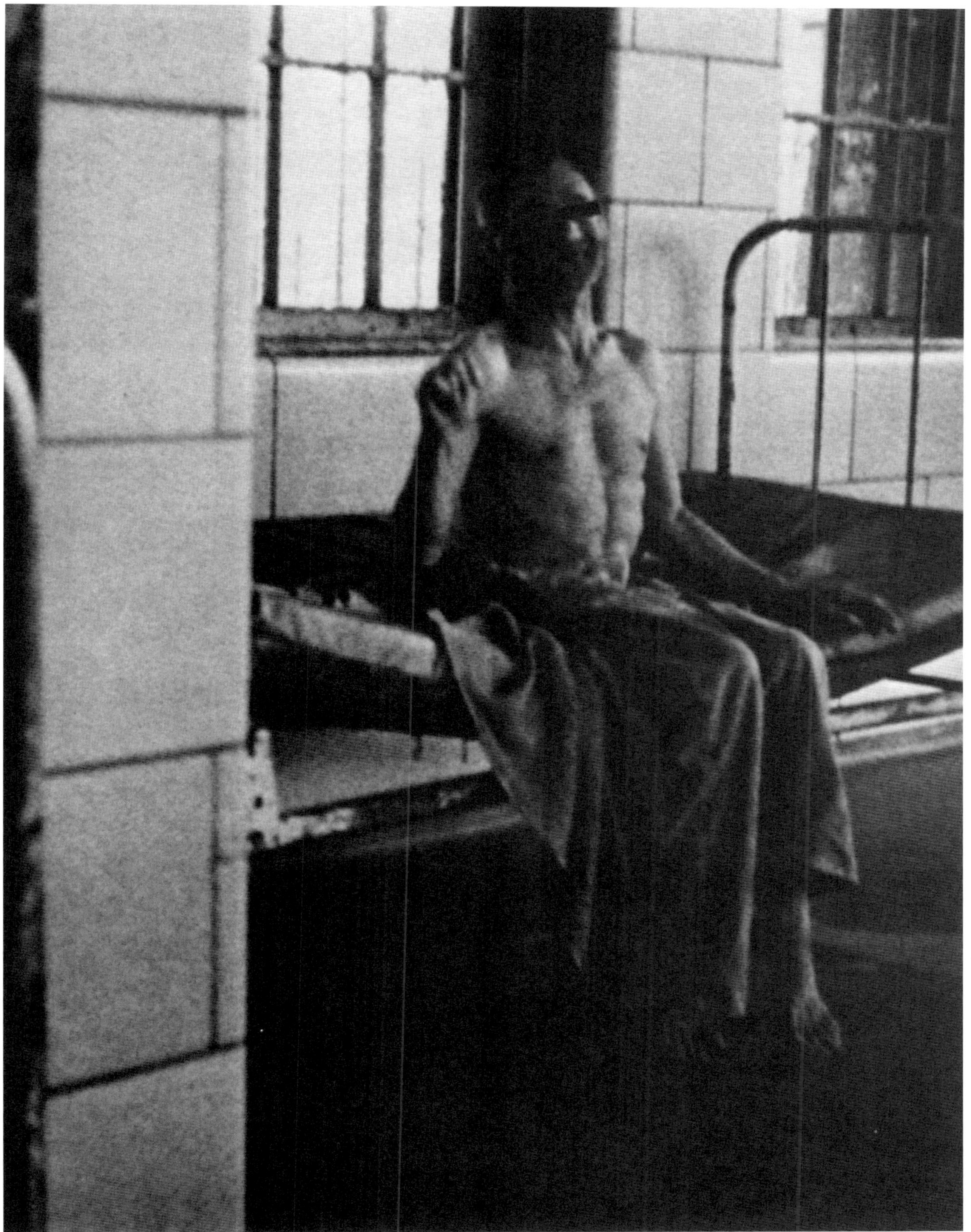

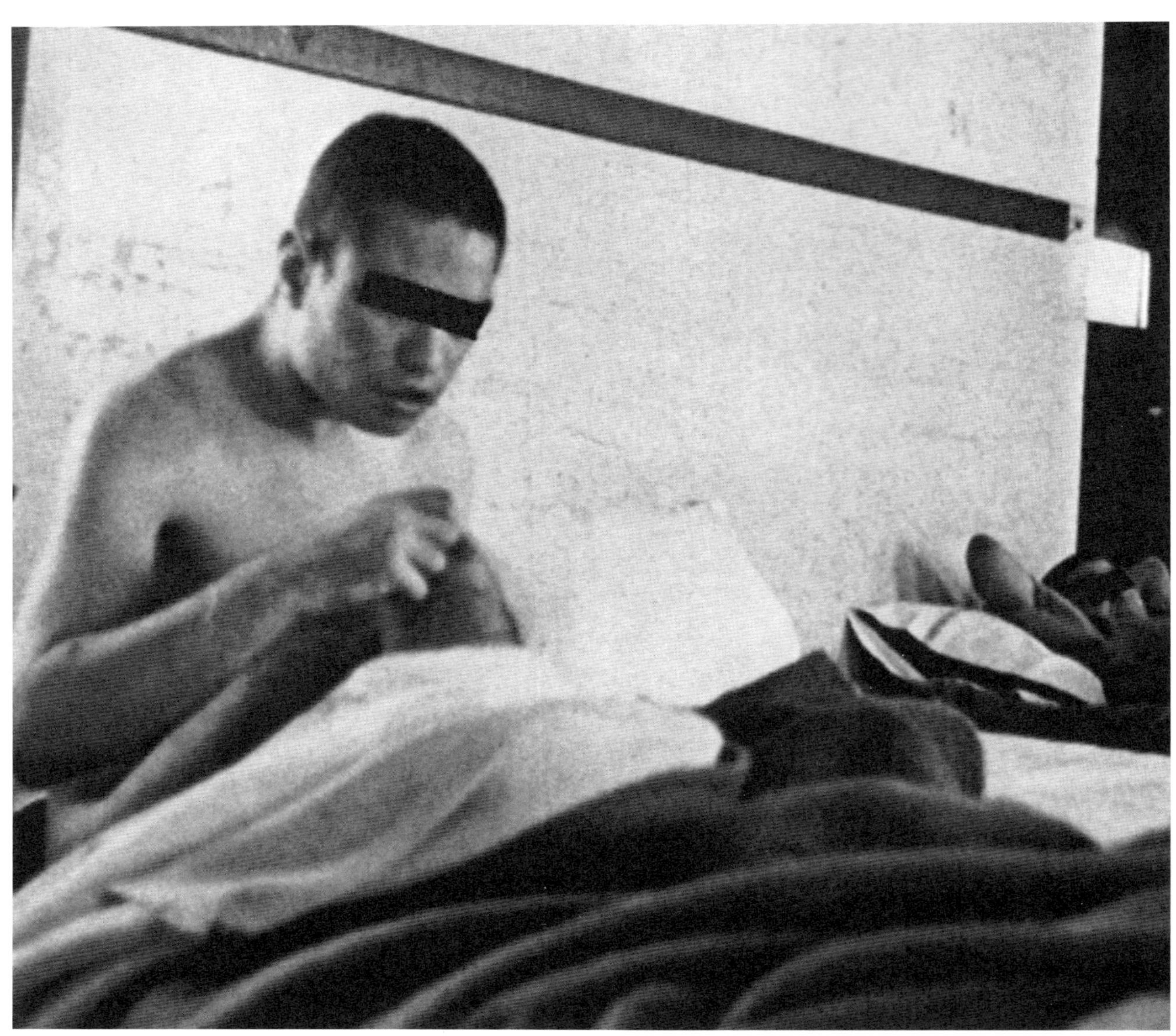

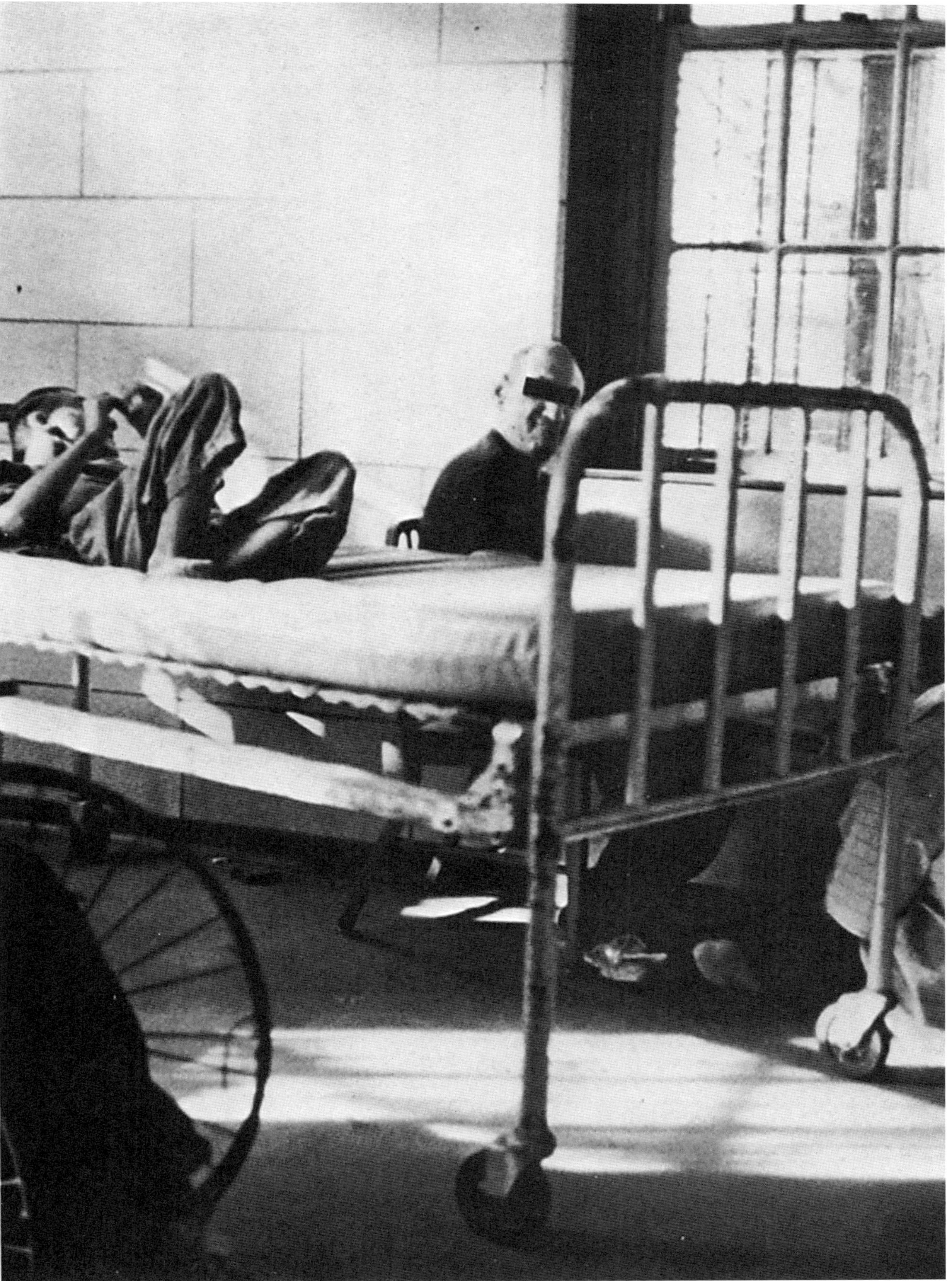

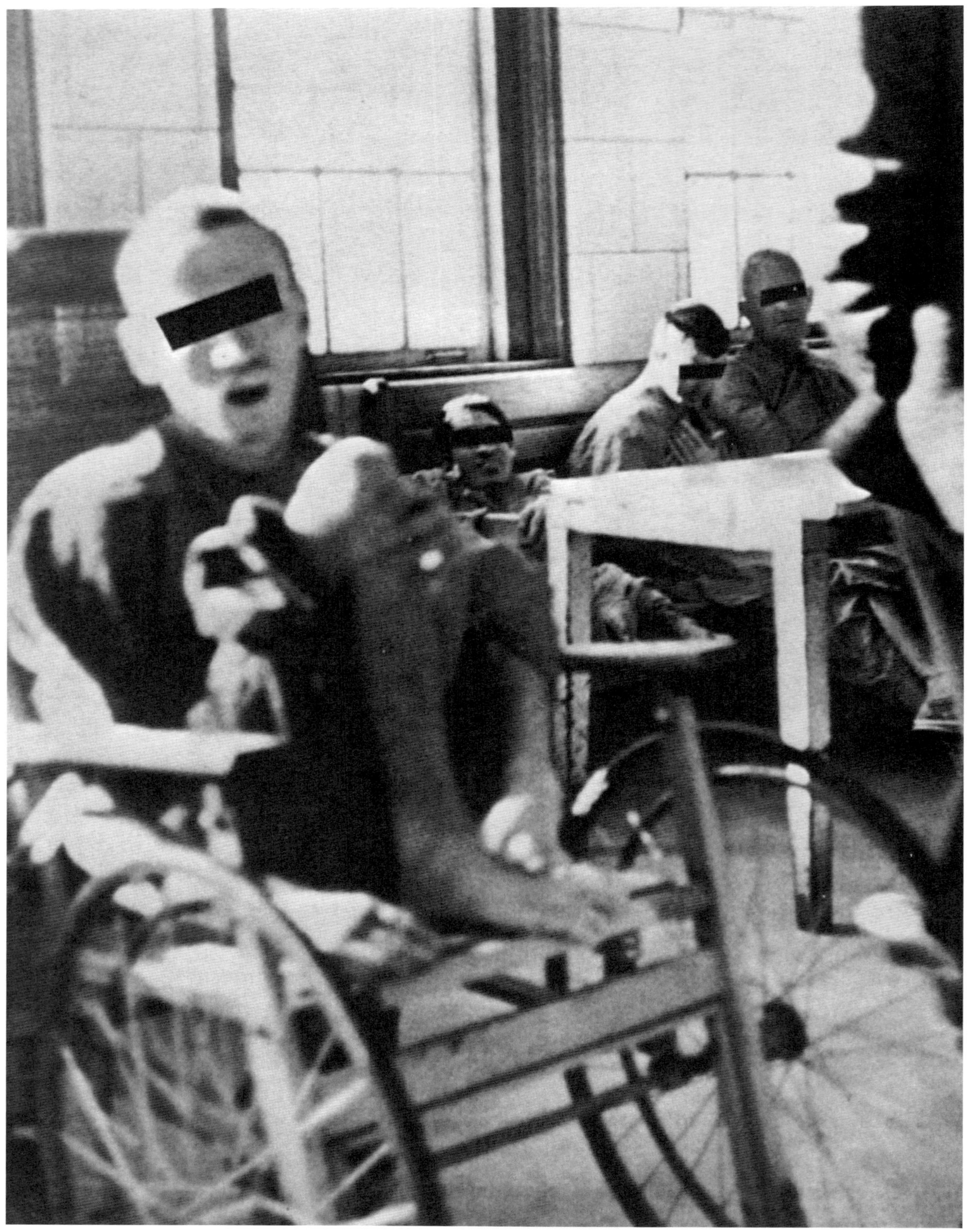

"Man is born into trouble, as the sparks fly upward."

Chronicles V, 7

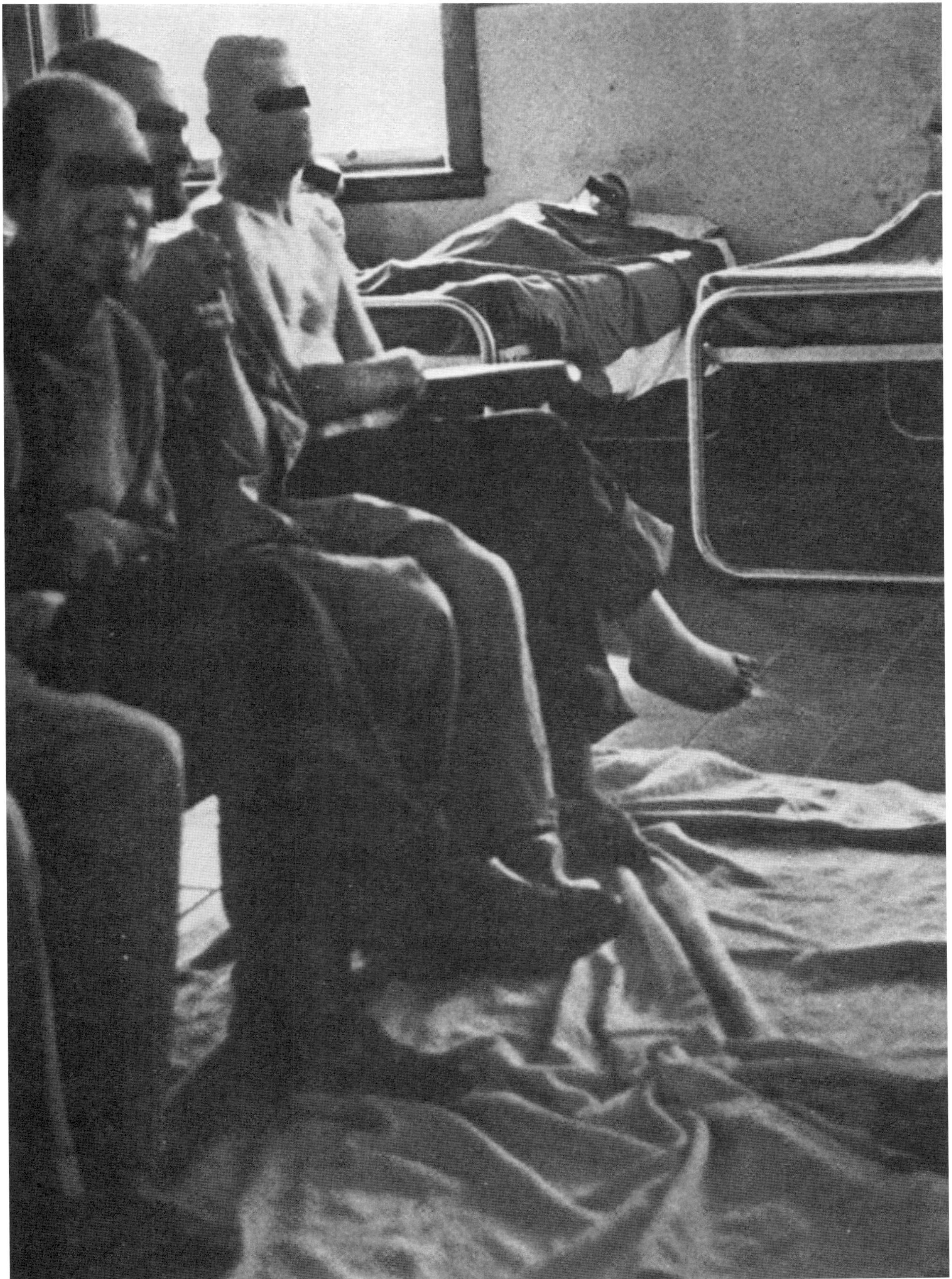

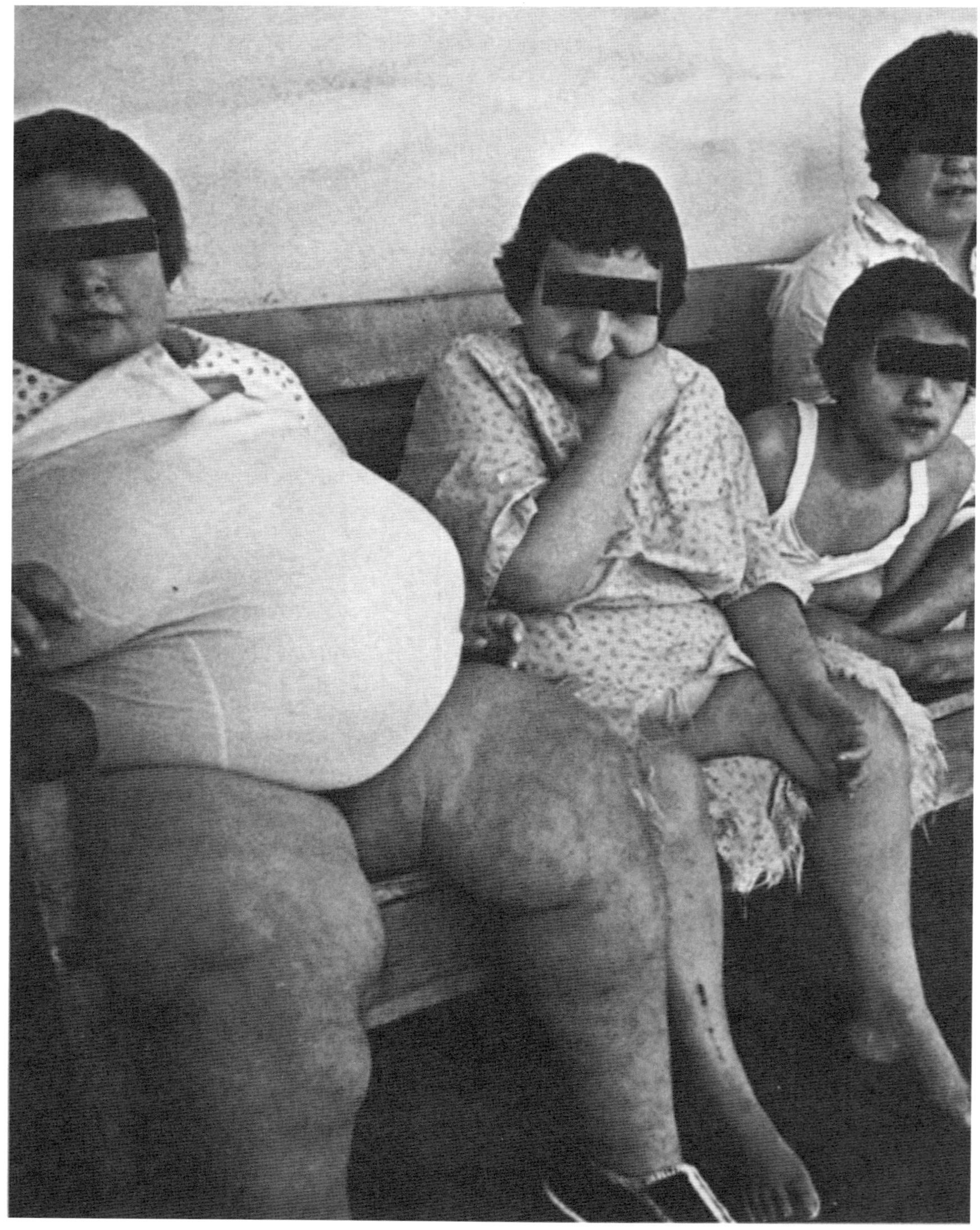

"Had I been present at the creation, I would have given some useful hints for the better ordering of the universe."

Alphonso the Learned

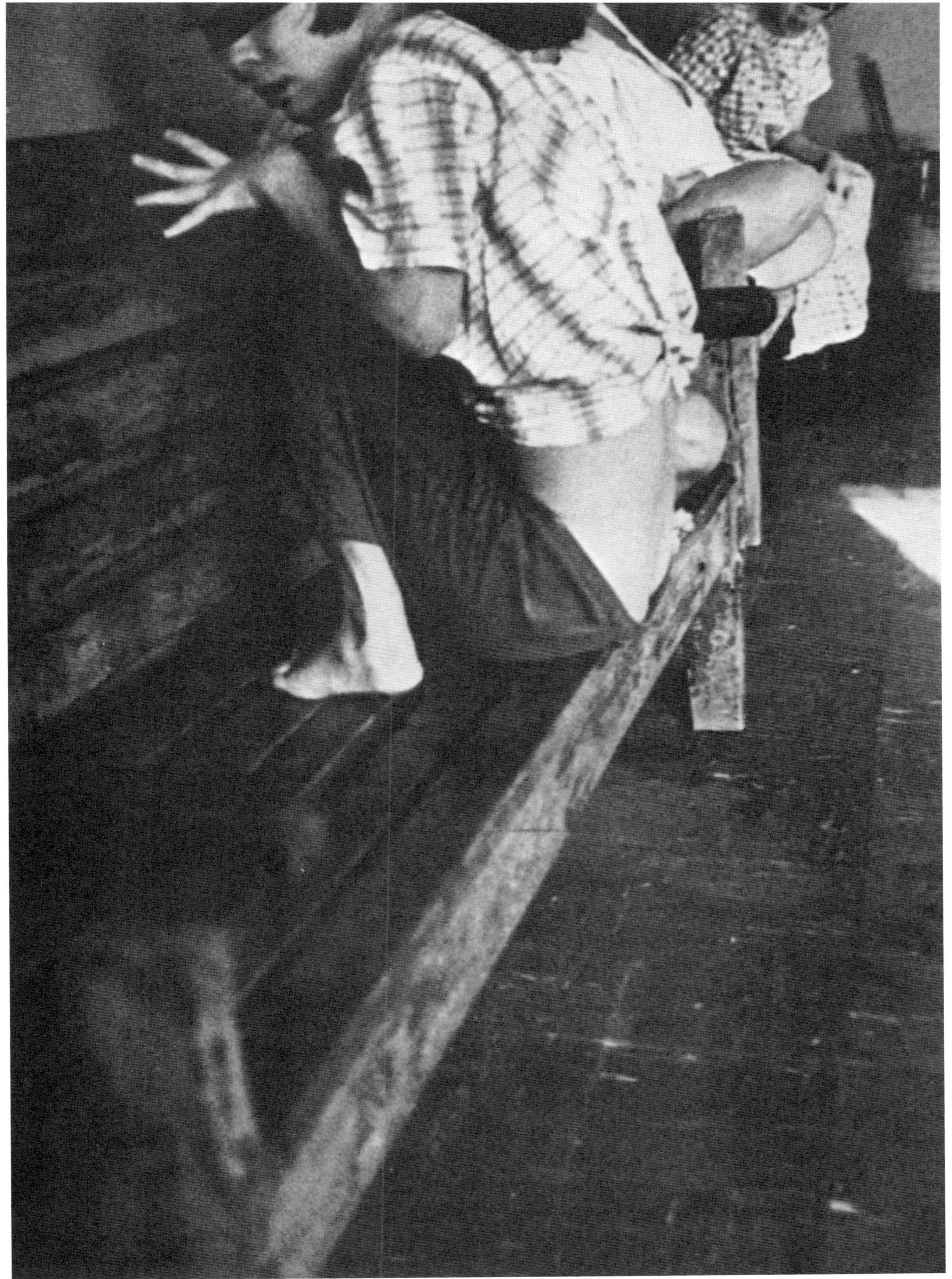

"In bed we laugh…"

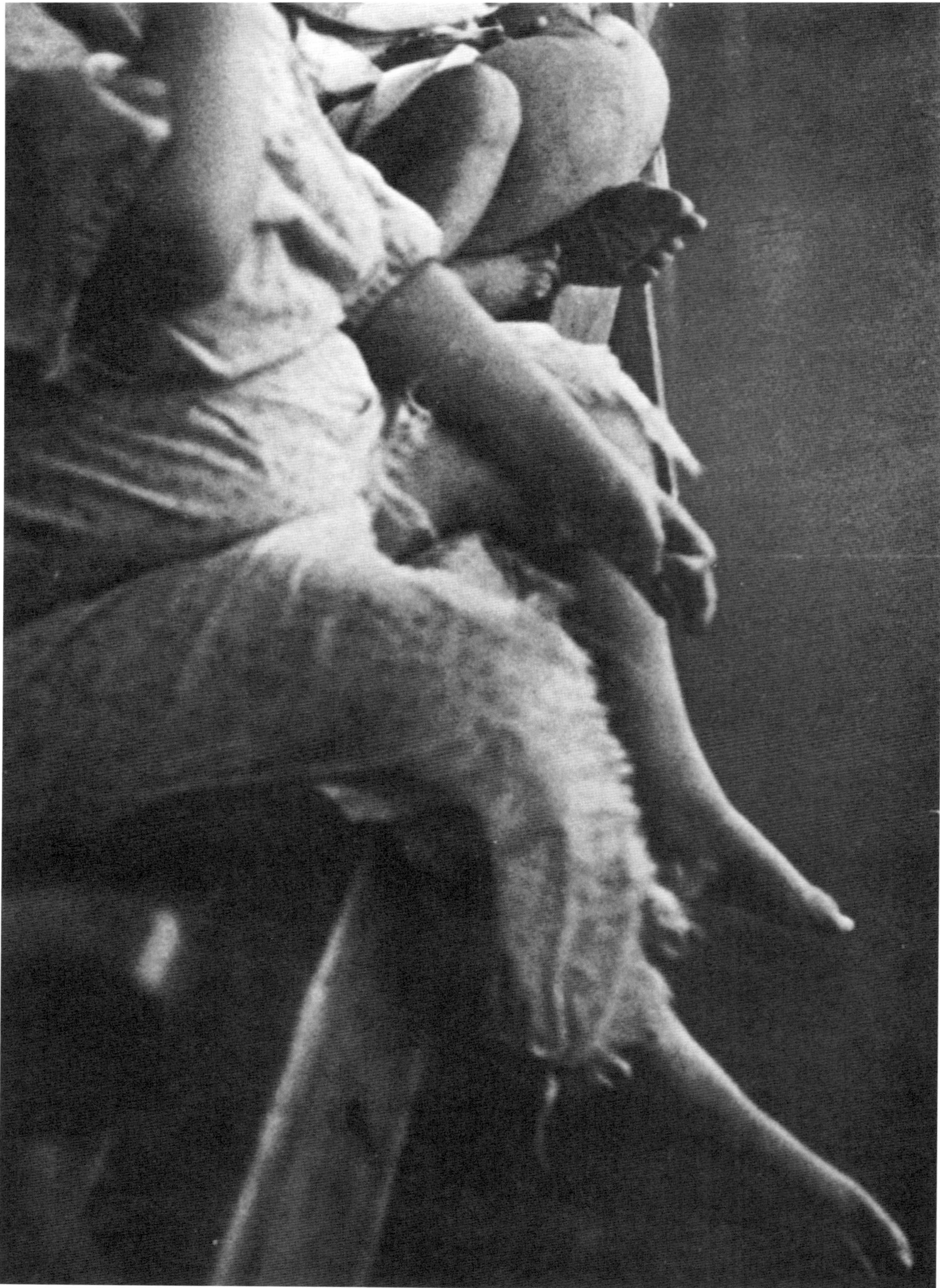

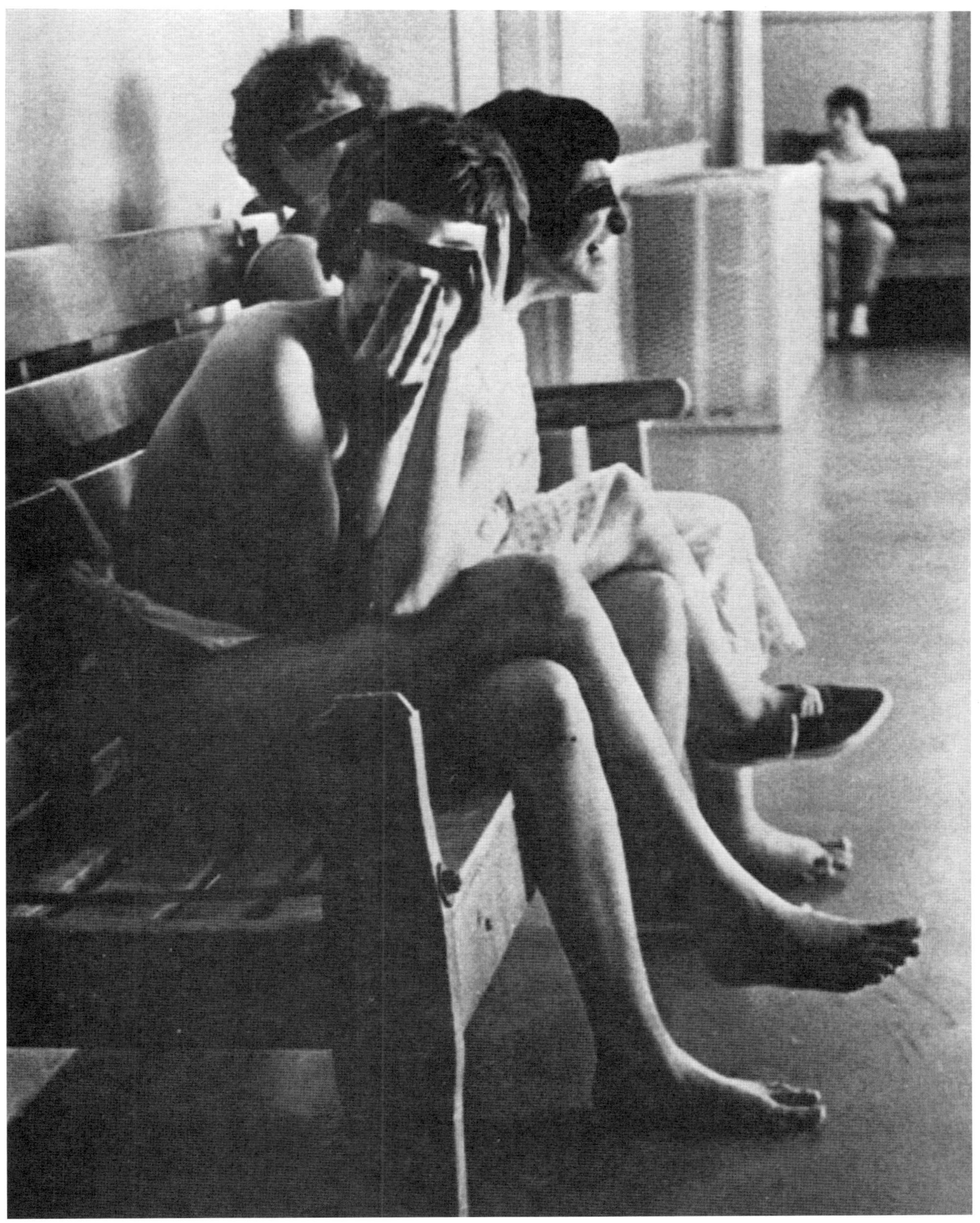

"I sometimes hold it half a sin to put in words the grief I feel."

Alfred, Lord Tennyson

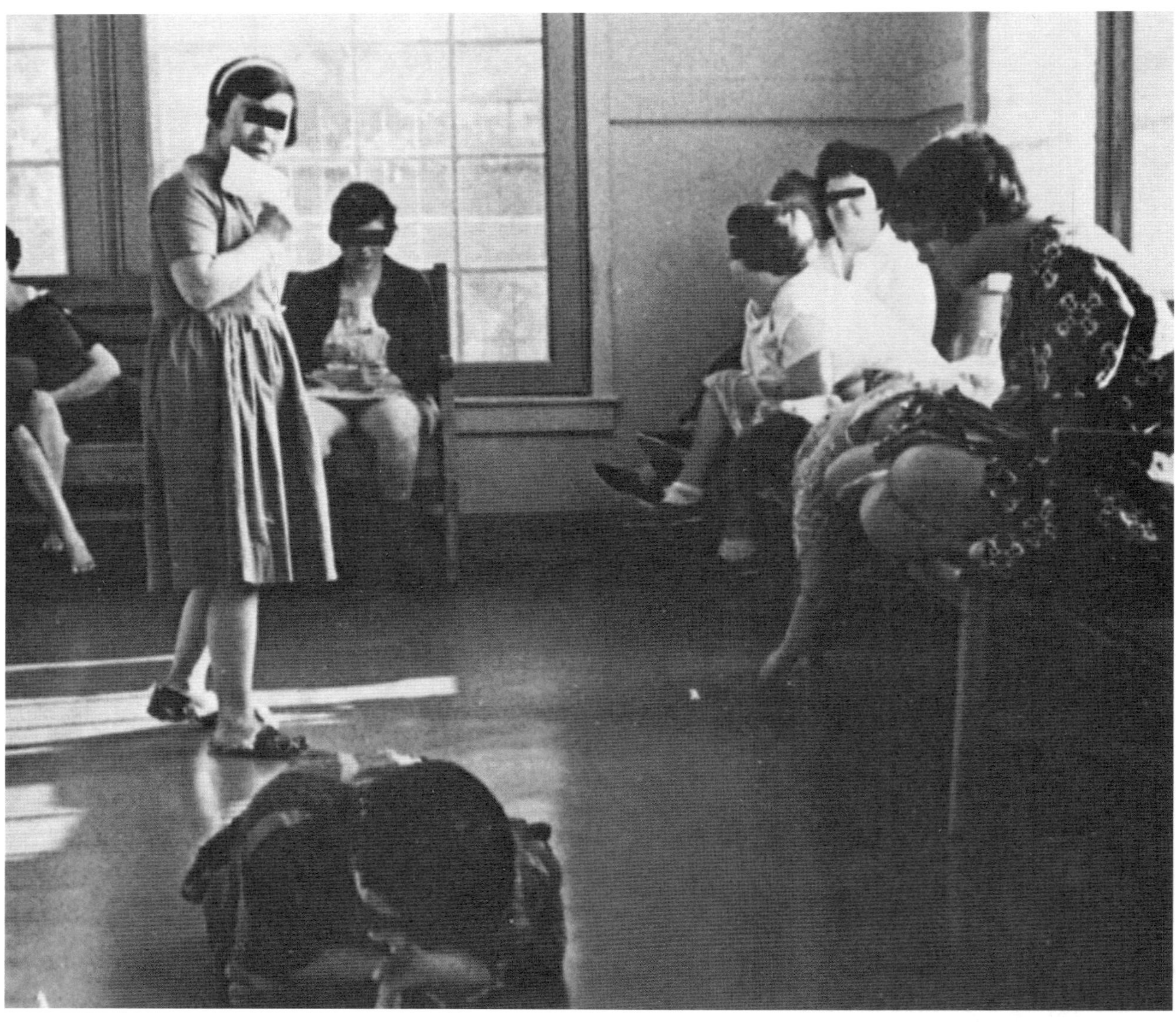

"A danger of early institutional training programs was their separateness from the reality of the outside world. This was something more than the poor personal habits—unhygenic, amoral, uncouth—which breed within walls. Rather it was the unconscious furthering of irresponsibility and provincialism. For conformity and withdrawal are the bulwarks of mass management; and both are alien to the rough-and-tumble world..."

Richard H. Hungerford

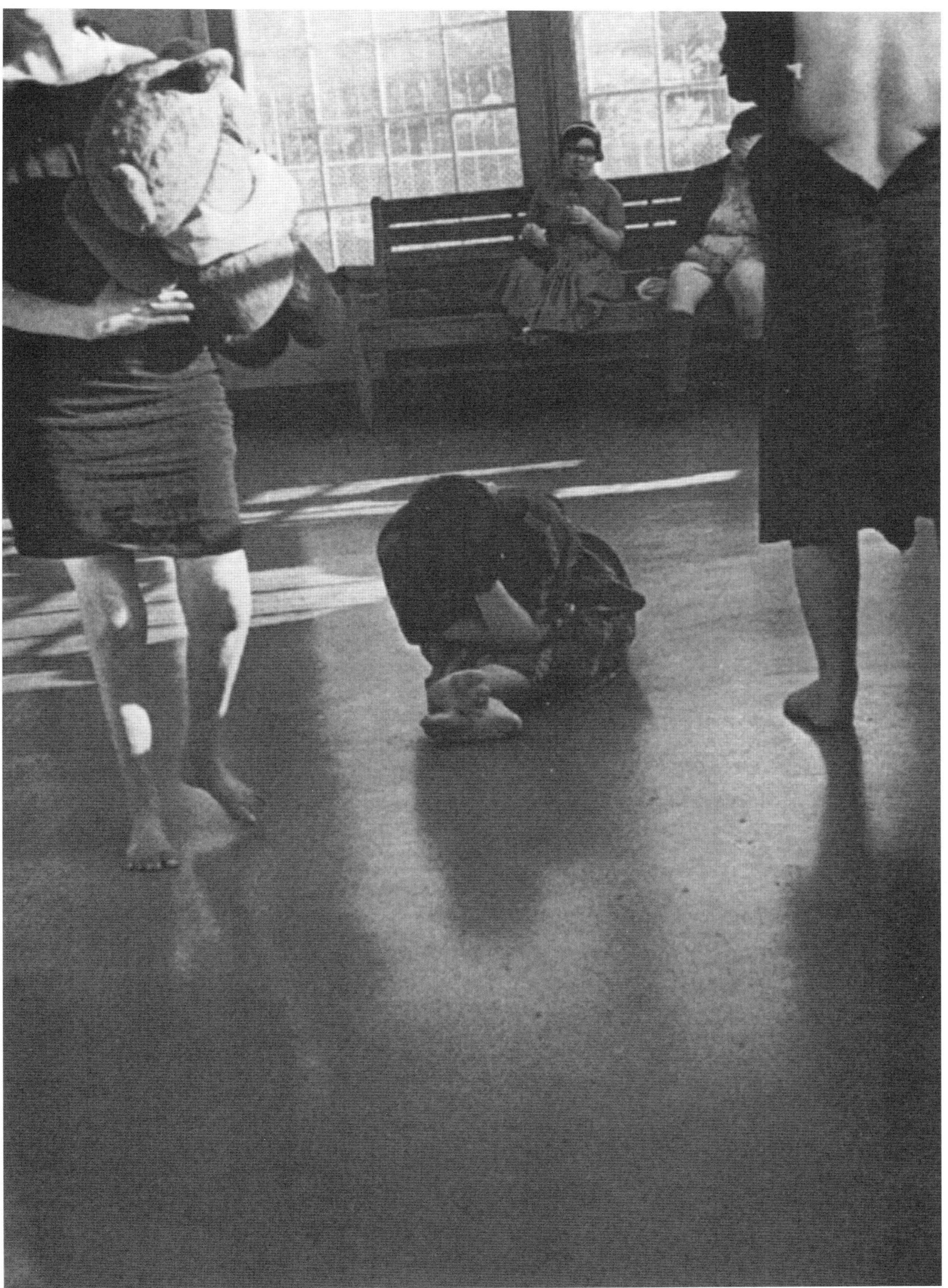

# Christmas in Purgatory

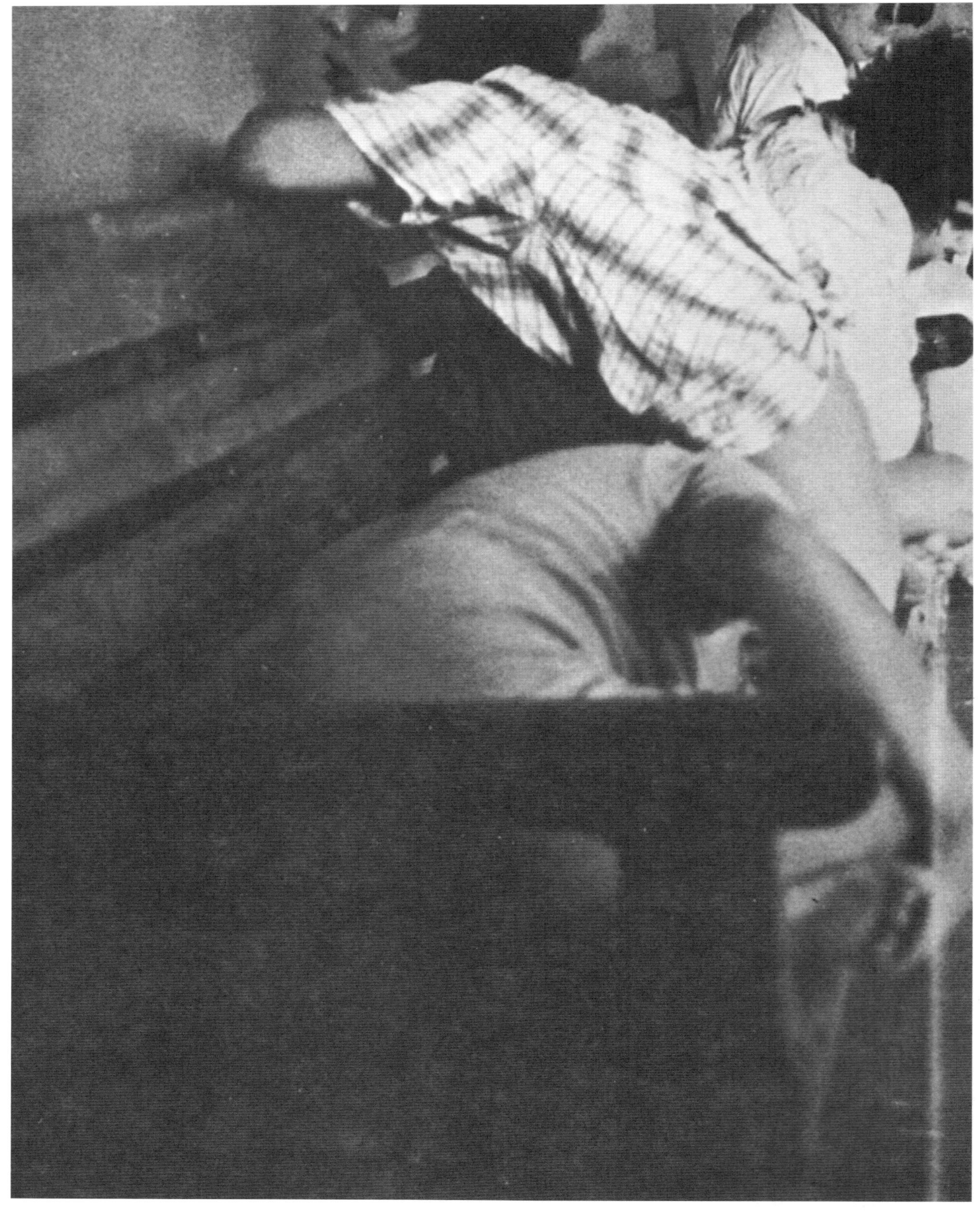

"One may find his religion in the clinical setting."

Albert T. Murphy

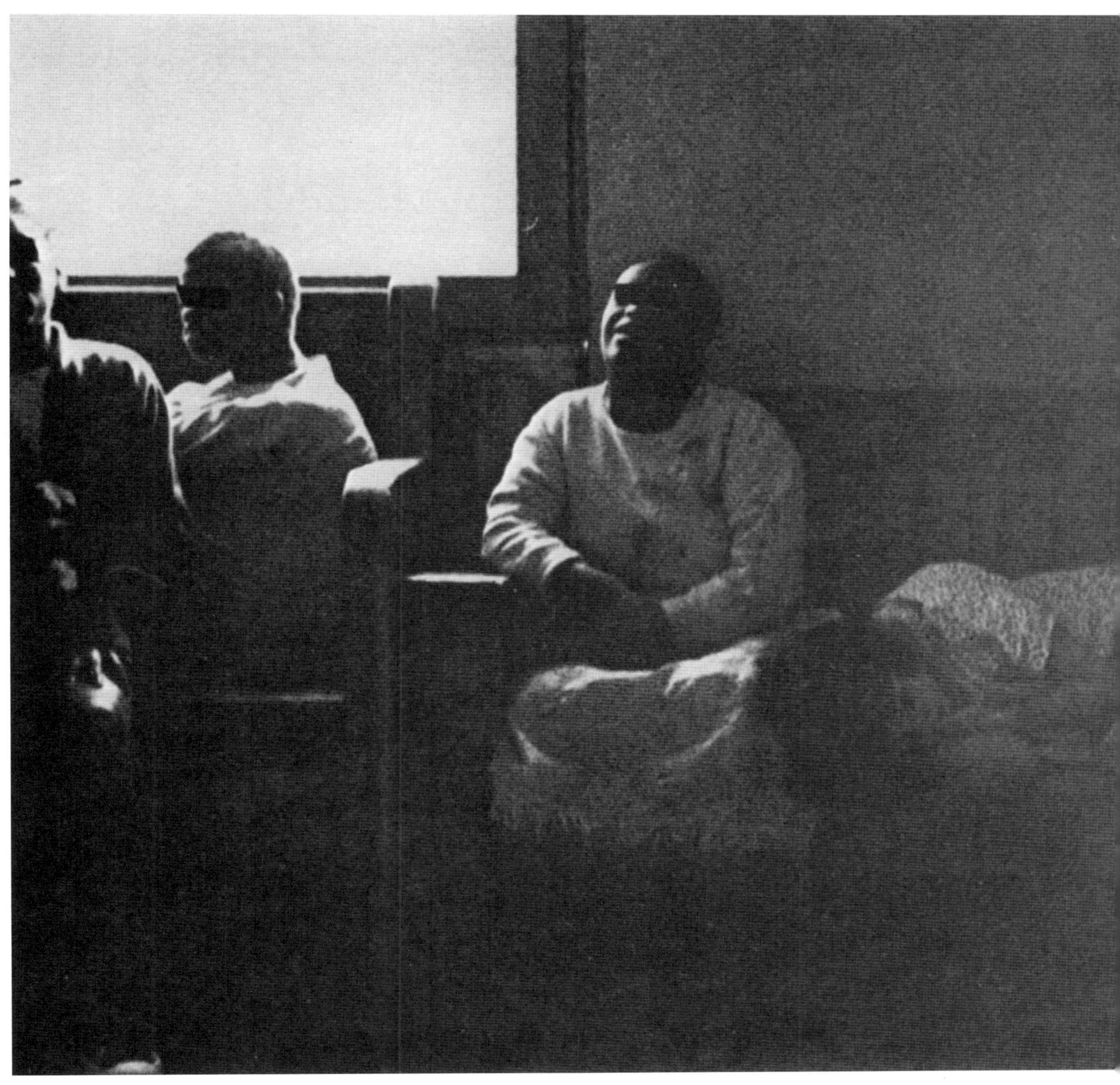

"Only the brave dare look upon the gray—upon the
things which cannot be explained easily, upon the
things which often engender mistakes, upon the
things whose cause cannot be understood..."

Richard H. Hungerford

# "The Promised Land..."

"The Promised Land always lies on the other side of a wilderness."

Havelock Ellis

About ten years ago, I made several trips to a large state institution for the mentally retarded, one not visited during the current study. I became interested in and, for several days, visited a dormitory housing severely retarded ambulatory adults—one that was very similar in population to those living quarters discussed in Part I. However, this dormitory was different in a very important way. What made this dormitory different can best be illustrated with the following story.

On the occasion of one such visit, I was hailed by one of the attendants and asked to come into the day room. The attendant called over a 35 or 40 year old, partly nude male and said, "Dr. Blatt, you remember Charlie. Charlie has learned how to say hello since your last visit. Charlie, say hello to Dr. Blatt." Charlie grunted and the attendant went into a kind of ecstasy that is rarely shown by adults and, when it is, radiates warmth for everyone lucky enough to be touched by it. It should not be misunderstood that Charlie's grunt resembled anything like a hello, or any other human utterance. In a way, this attendant's reaction to Charlie might have been considered as a kind of psychopathology of its own. However, we have a different understanding of it.

What kind of man was this attendant? In 1938 he walked, literally off the streets, into that institution—an alcoholic, without a home of his own, purposeless and without a future—and asked for a job. For twenty-eight years he has served as an attendant in a dormitory for severely retarded patients at this institution. He knows every "boy" there and actually thinks of them as his children and they of him as their father.

Sometimes, in despair and helplessness, we ask ourselves why were these severely retarded human beings born. When one observes an attendant of the kind we have just described, it is possible to find an answer. If not for the mentally retarded this attendant might have been a drifter, an alcoholic, much less of a person than he actually is. Would it be unfair to say that this attendant needed mental retardation in order to fulfill his own destiny and obtain the greatest good he could render to society?

Mental retardation can bring out the best in some people—as well as the worst. At The Seaside, it brings out the best in a lot of different adults who are involved professionally, interpersonally, and tangentially, with the residents. The Seaside has more of the people of the kind we have just discussed, than do other places for the mentally retarded—notwithstanding the fact that every institution, large as well as small and those discussed in Part I as well as The Seaside, has superb and dedicated attendants and professional staff as well as its quota of mediocre and poor staff. In our opinion, The Seaside has more superior personnel and fewer of the inefficient and disinterested. We believe this is a major difference between The Seaside and other institutions for the mentally retarded.

The following portion of a report, written by a Seaside nursery teacher, concerning a child with whom she is working speaks volumes about such matters as clinical sensitivity, thoughtfulness, and the value one human being is capable of placing on another. The investment and dedication of one person to another is the significant history of any case study illustrating behavioral change:

> She came into our Day-Care a fiery haired five-year old with a temper the same shade. Cerebral palsied, and unable to talk, she lashed out at unfair world with an unspeakable fury. Torn by the mixed emotions of her parents who had alternately spoiled and dis-

ciplined her, this extremely sensitive child seemed beyond control when she entered our little group. The hurricane raged for several weeks when I probed all the re cesses of my mind to find the eye of the storm. We learned to duck with agility all that she threw, to keep a level head, and to follow, with the strictest adherence, a routine designed for the comfort and growth of all the children. We ignored her nonconformities. Her actions, for all intents and purposes, were not getting through to me. Furthermore, they were not impressing her classmates.

All this time she watched me. She wanted me to be angry too for this was her trick in trade. Oh how I wanted to spank her for her tirades and inconsiderations but I did not because this procedure would be old hat to her.

One day I was particularly tired and discouraged and she must have sensed something amiss. Spilling milk is not unusual in a pre-school situation, but our little firebrand made a last stand. She threw her milk at me with deadly accuracy. I sat stunned for a minute. As the milk dripped from my hair, I deliberated—one false move could undo everything. I felt an angry tear in my eye. She looked at me, her face red and contorted with emotion. I didn't move. Suddenly, she staggered from the room. Still I sat, knowing I must take some action. A few moments passed. She came running back into the room, hands dripping with wet paper towels. I didn't move. She smoothed back my hair and wiped my face and clothes with erratic, awkward hands. She had suddenly dissolved into a compassion she failed to comprehend because she had never needed it; it was a brand new experience. Involuntarily my arms went out and she flew in.

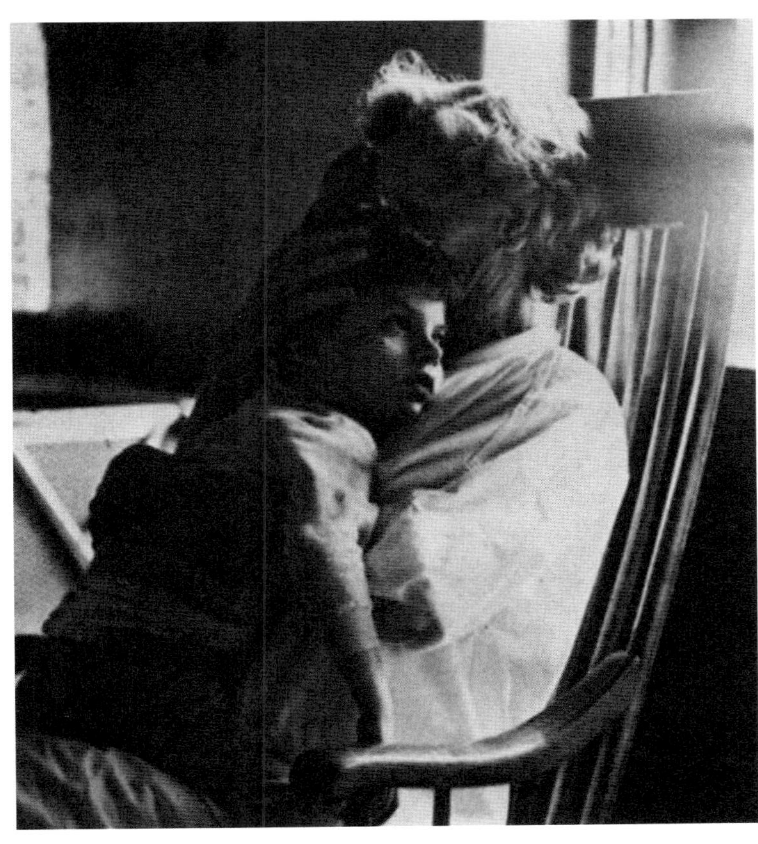

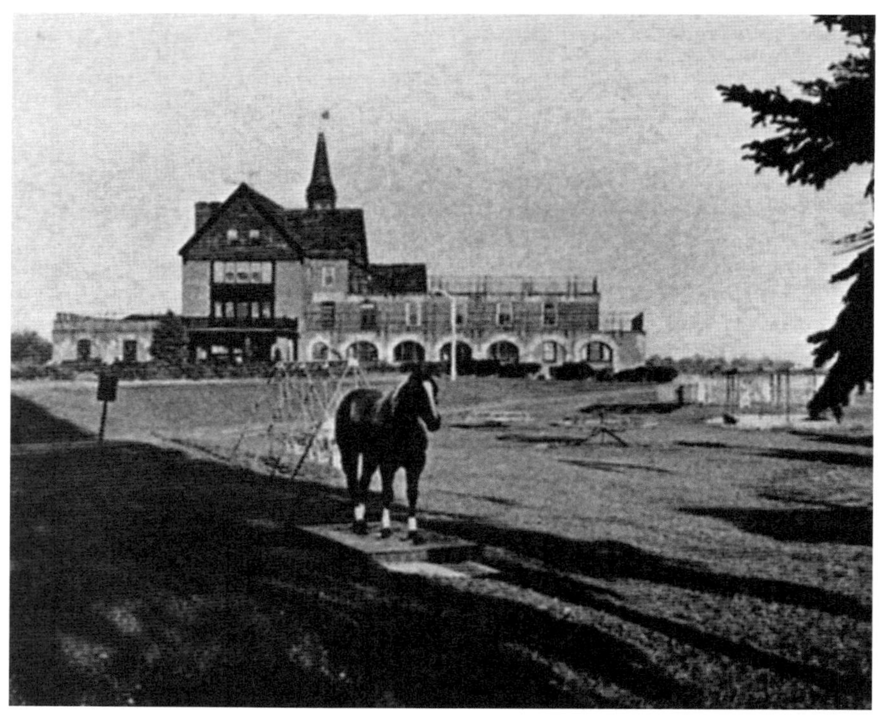

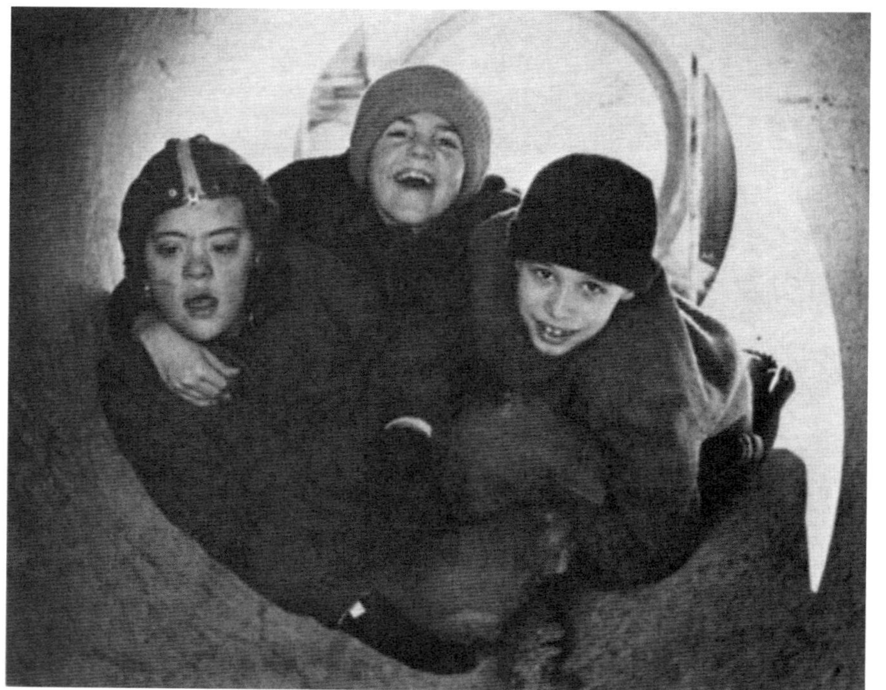

"The mentally retarded continue to be the least of the last minority in the United States— the least understood, the most different, the least appreciated. Still it seems probable that, in the words of Voltaire, 'Their time has come.' And, in spite of the ignorance and general indifference of the public, the lot of the retarded is looking upward."

Richard H. Hungerford

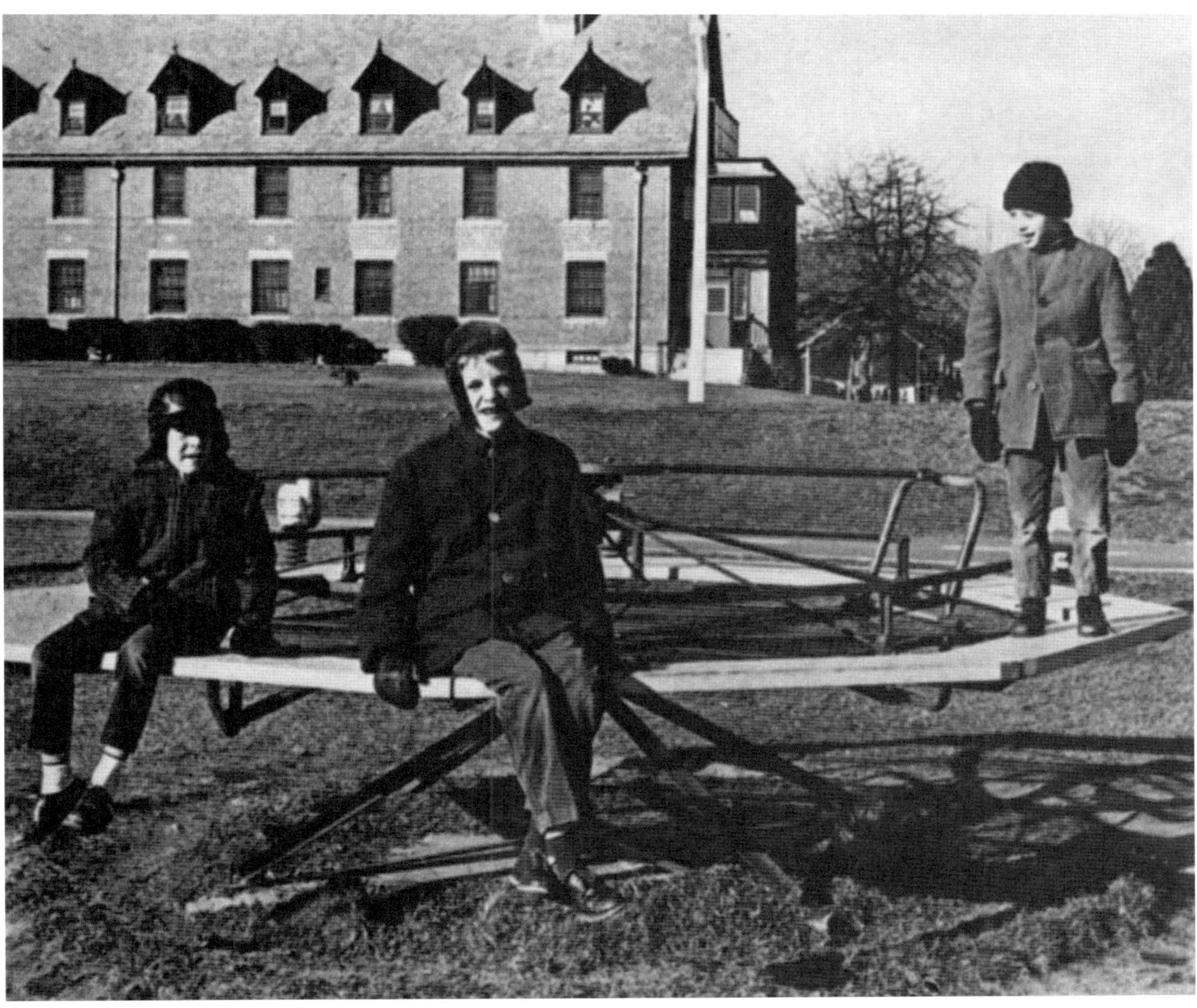

"Cultural and educational deprivation resulting in mental retardation can also be prevented."

John Fitzgerald Kennedy

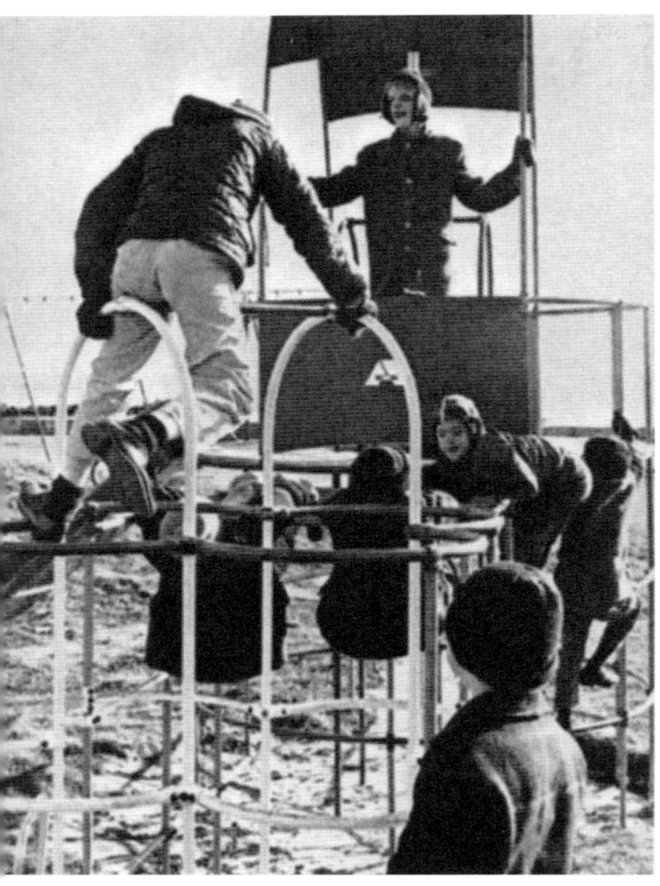

"Can we ever have too much of a good thing?"

Miguel de Cervantes

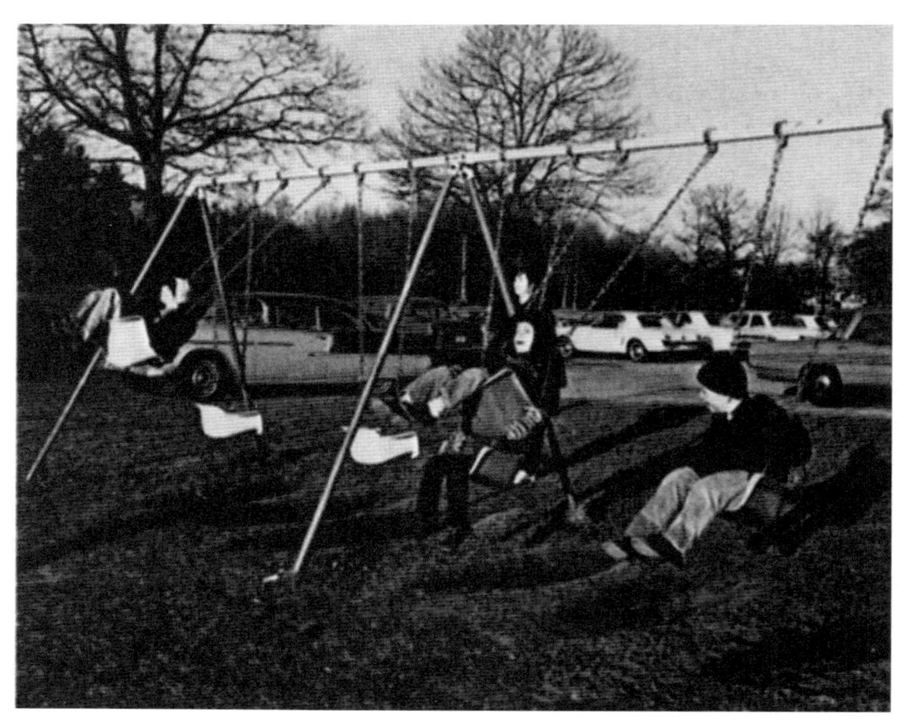

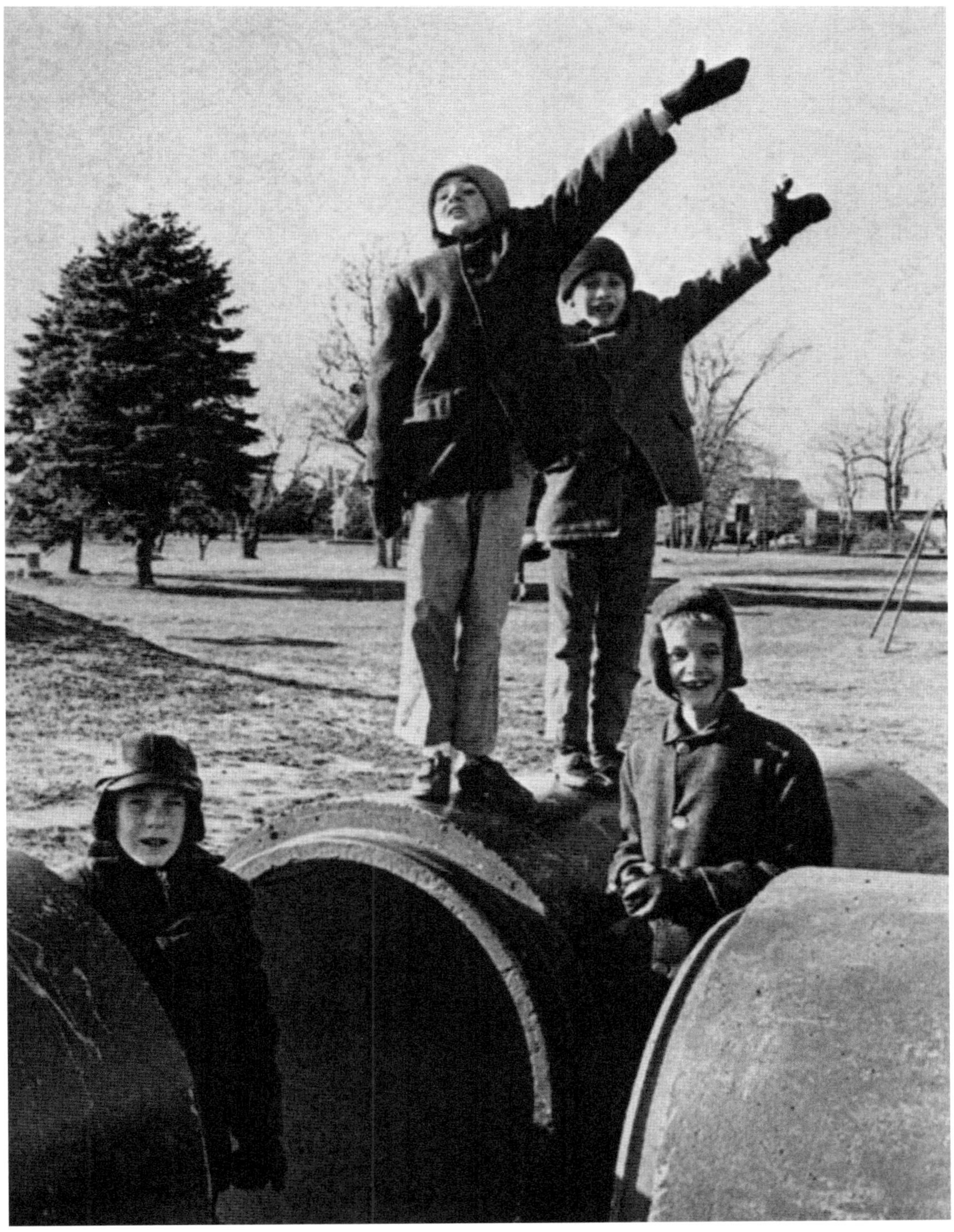

"What would man be without Utopia? He must aim at the unattainable in order to realize the attainable and to make one step forward."

Thomas Mann

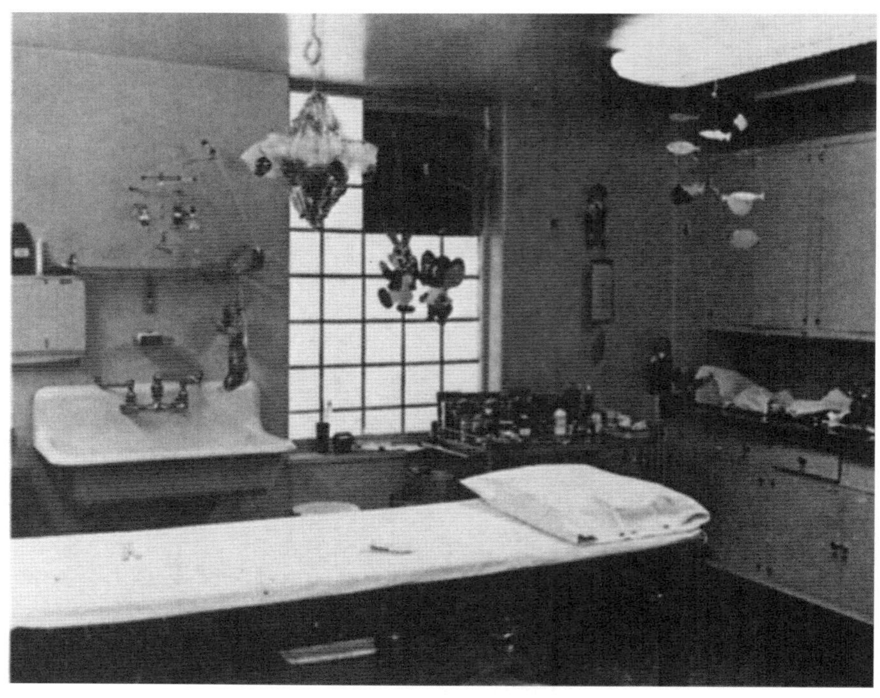

"The wheels of humanitarianism never grind as fast as when they are aided by utilitarianism."

Richard H. Hungerford

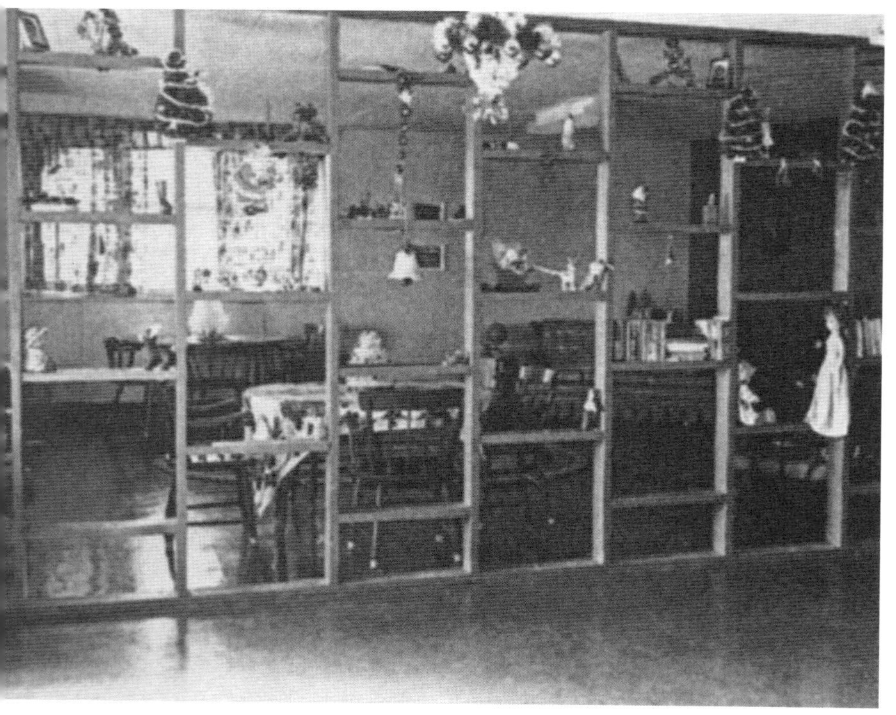

"At Christmas play and make good cheer
For Christmas comes but once a year."

Thomas Tusser

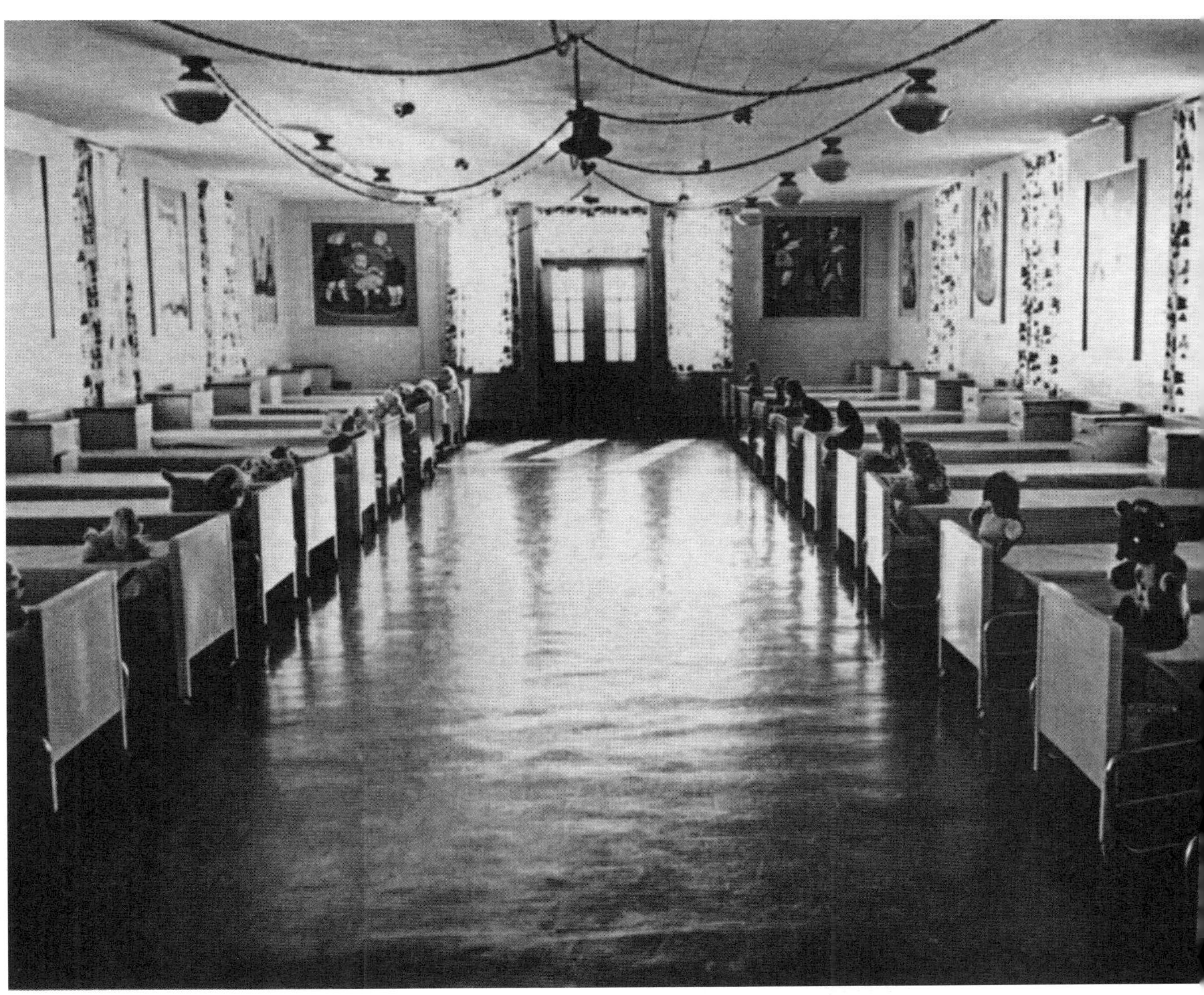

"During the eighteenth century the plight of the mentally ill was shocking almost everywhere in Europe. …flighty, troublesome or dangerous patients were restrained and kept in a small room or stall in a private house, in 'lunatic boxes,' in cages or in other places of confinement that seemed appropriate for isolating them and rendering them harmless…as a result of poor supervision, many committed suicide, perished through accidents or created serious disturbances. The tense and exasperating environment thus created and encouraged the establishment of the strictest preventative measures."

Emil Kraepelin

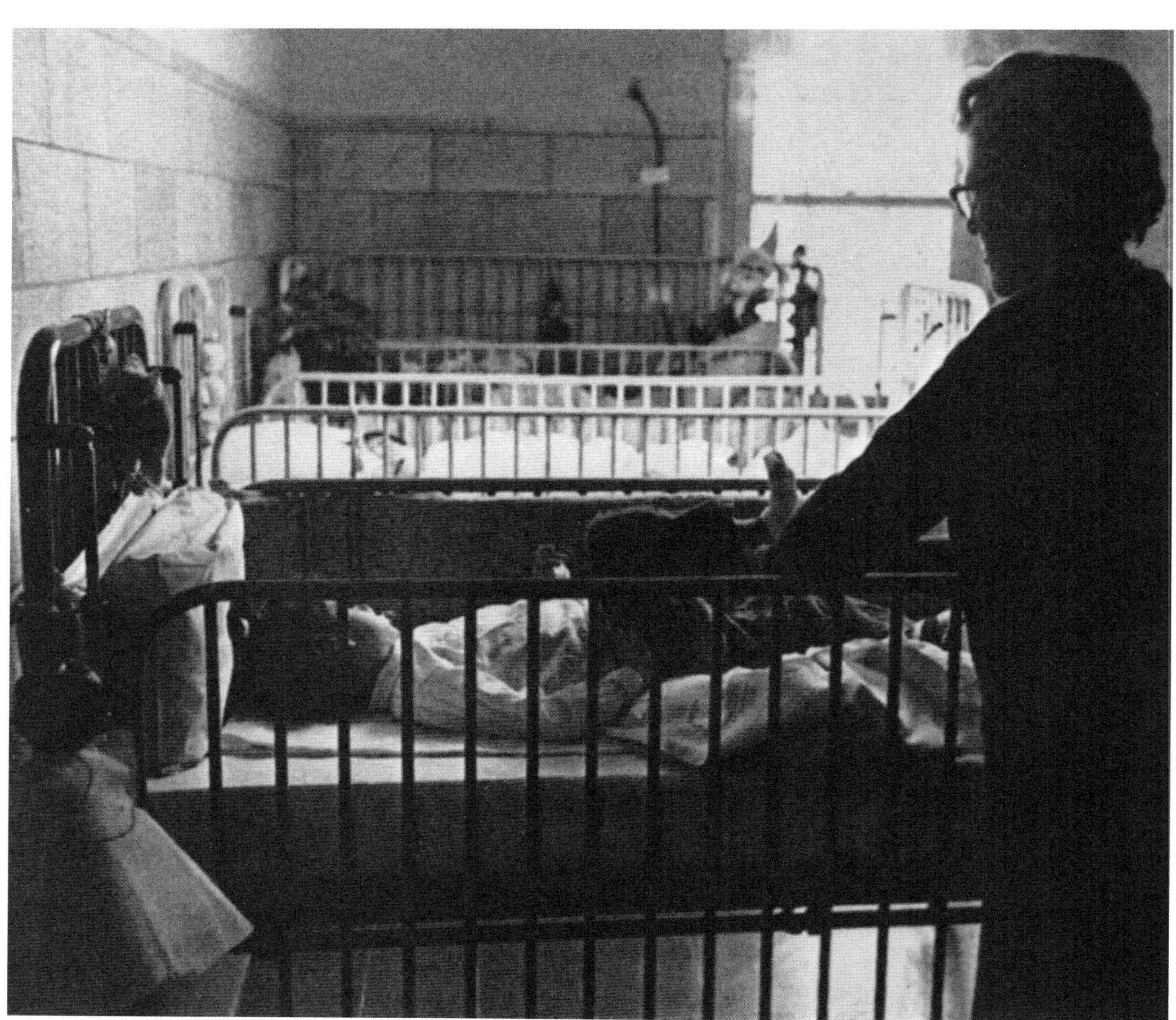

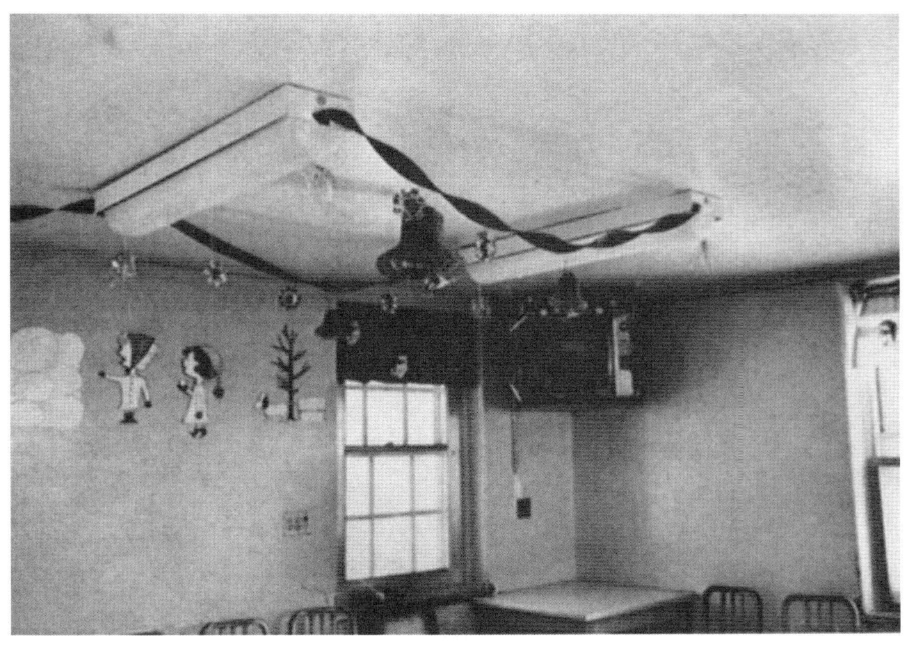

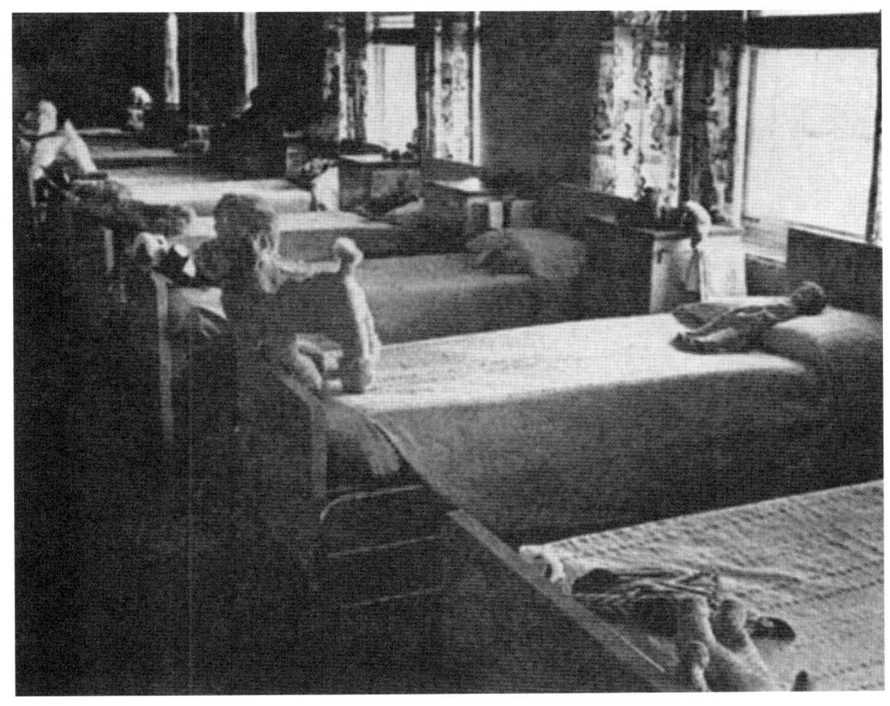

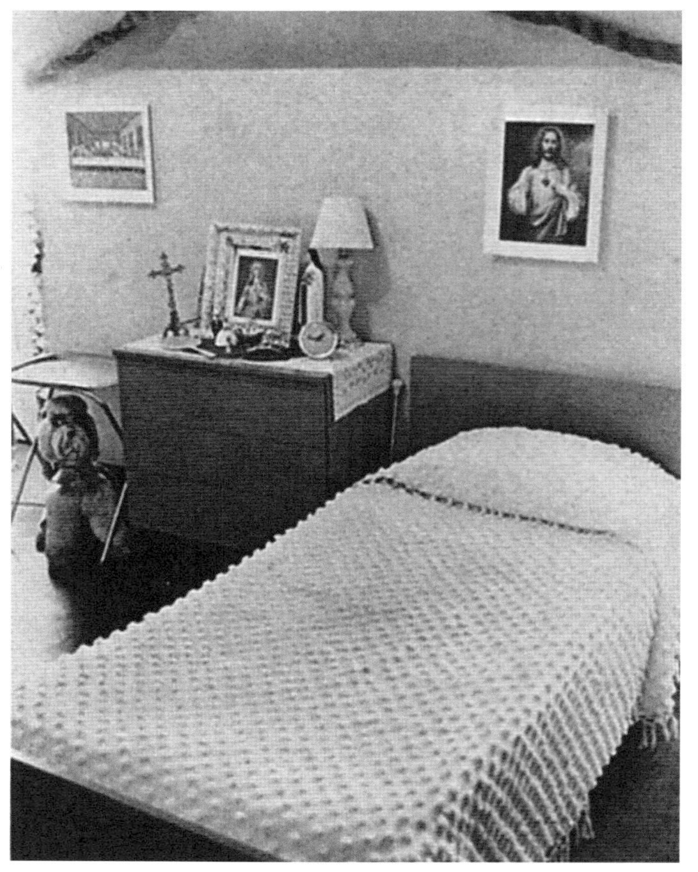

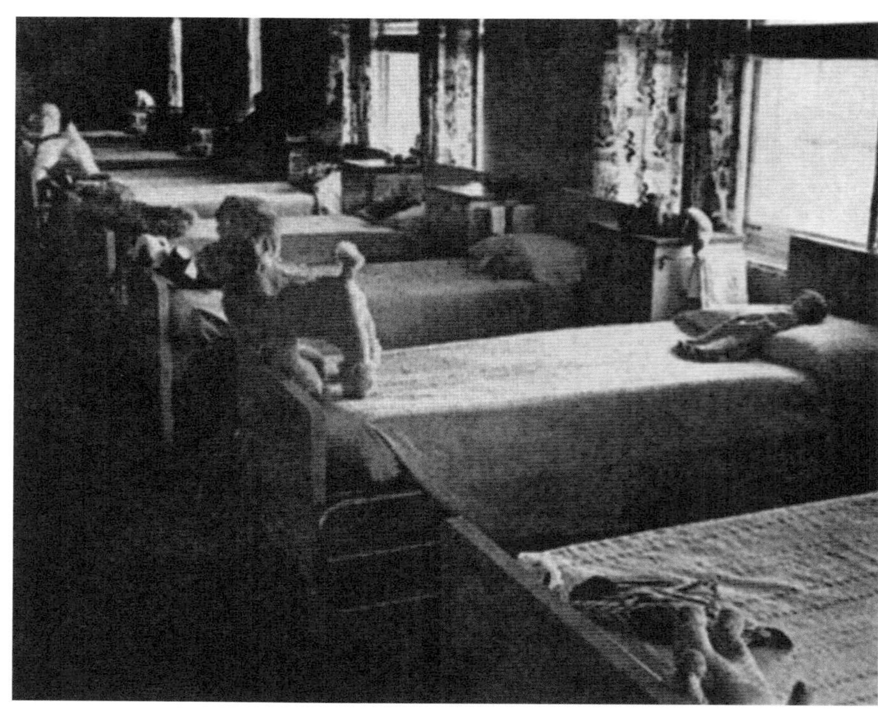

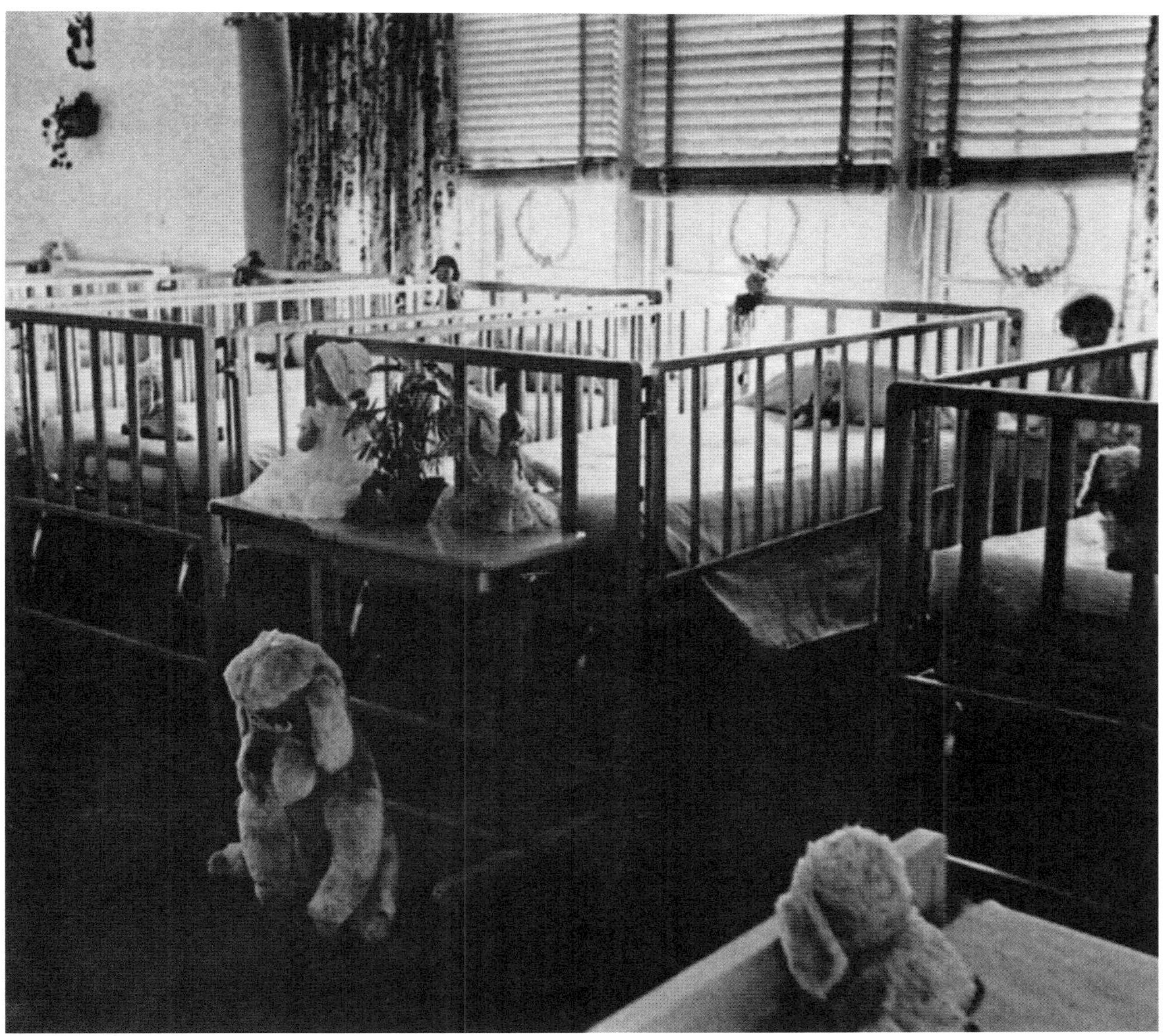

"Those who visited Bedlam in London in 1814 could see countless patients clad only in loose shrouds and chained by their arms or legs to the wall in such a way that they could stand upright or remain seated. One patient for 12 years wore rings around his neck and waist and was tethered to a wall; because he had resisted attempts to control his movements by means of a chain manipulated from a neighboring room, the warden had also taken the precaution of lashing his arms to his sides. An administrator explained that chains were the surest device for restraining recalcitrant mental patients. Even Dr. Monro stated in response to an investigating committee of the House of Commons that no one dared to use chains on noblemen, but that they were indispensable in dealing with the poor and those in public institutions."

Emil Kraepelin

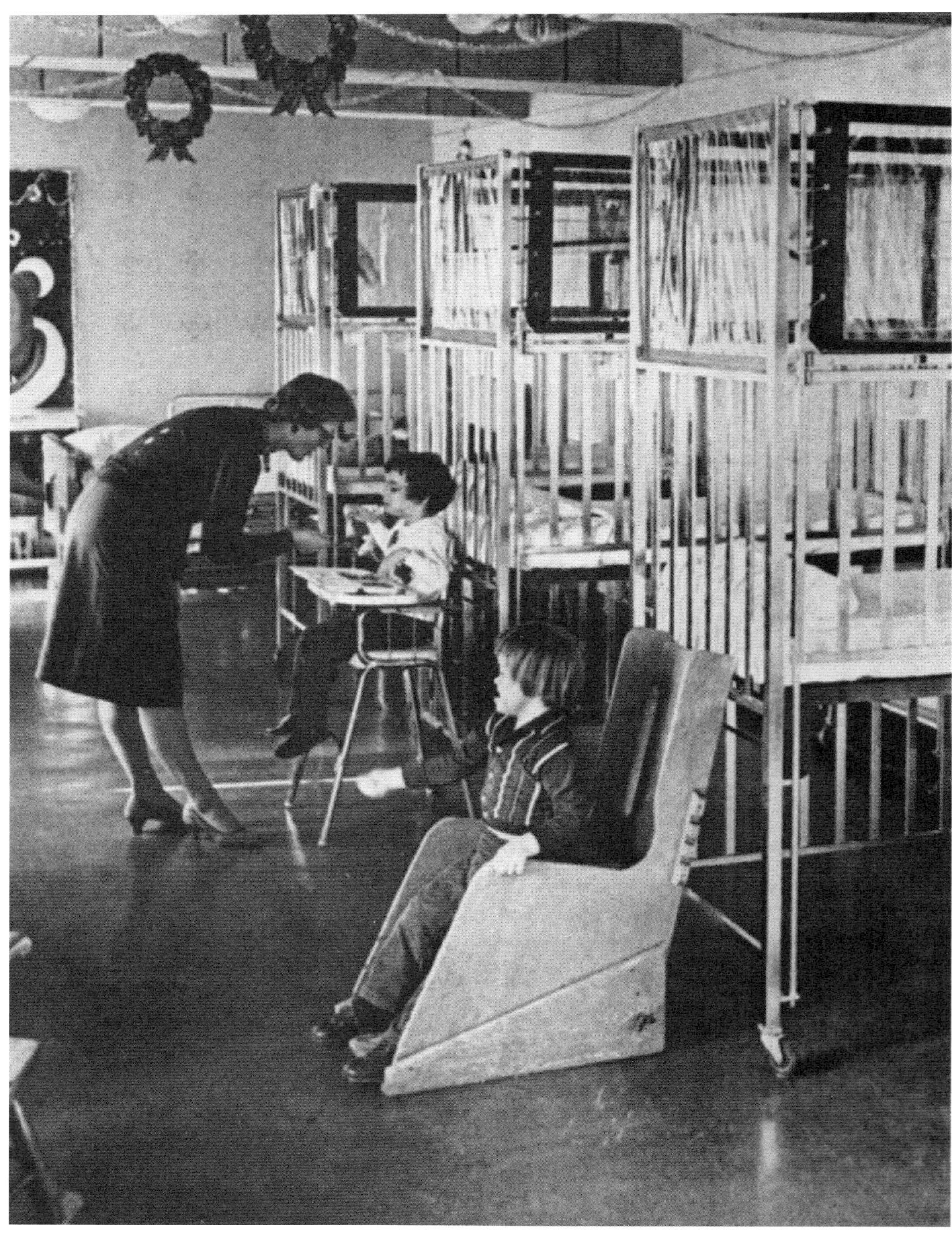

"Have you had a kindness shown?
Pass it on."

Henry Burton

# "We have developed a myth…"

"We have developed a myth revolving about the specialness of our curricula efforts to date. In some important ways, there is as great a myth concerning the specialness of the children the curricula seek to serve."

During one visit to a large state institution discussed in Part I, we were told about the development of a new research center on the institutional grounds. The assistant superintendent mentioned to us that the "materials" for the research center would come from the institution and this center would require the addition of approximately 30 or 40 "items." We were confused by the statement and, as a result of some verbal fumbling and embarrassment, we finally understood. At that institution, and apparently at others in that state, patients are called "material" and personnel are called "items."

It was so difficult not to believe that this assistant superintendent was "pulling our leg" with his terminology that during our subsequent visits to dormitories in that institution we asked the attending physician "How many items do you having in this building? How much material do you have?" To our amazement, he knew exactly what we were asking for and gave us the numbers immediately.

The Seaside does not deal with "material" and "items." The Seaside is a small institution of approximately 250 residents and somewhat over 100 staff. As importantly, the Center services the community where it is located. Many children and adults living at home with their families attend pre-school classes, recreation groups, sheltered workshops, and other activities sponsored by the institution.

The uniqueness of The Seaside results from an extraordinarily dedicated and involved staff in a setting small enough for every child-care worker—as well as every teacher, nurse, and administrator—to know each child in the institution and vice versa.

At The Seaside, there is time, time for teaching a young child to use a spoon or fork, time for helping a child learn to use a zipper, time to heal a wound—physical or emotional. But there is no time for tomorrow at The Seaside. There is a fight against inertia. Children must be helped today, for in too few tomorrows children become adults and residents become inmates.

At The Seaside there is schooling. Some children attend school at the institution. The older and more capable youngsters attend public schools—with other children who are living at home. The environment is designed for children. The lawns are filled with swings and jungle gyms and bicycle paths. During Christmastime, each room is decorated welcoming Santa Claus and the spirit of Christmas. Rooms are clean and orderly. Furniture is designed for children. Furniture for adults is designed for adults.

There are adults residents at The Seaside, but not in the same dormitories, and programs for adults are also separate. Adults have different needs and the following may illustrate how some of these are met.

One of our difficulties in photographing activities at The Seaside was our inability to take very many pictures of adult residents. Most of the adults at The Seaside are working during the day, on institutional jobs or out in the community. Some, who could not be returned to their own homes, live in a work training unit. Here they are friends and co-workers under the careful supervision of a cottage mother and father. During the day they are on placement—working in the community—and in the evening they return to their "home" where they can receive special help and guidance in their successful attempts to integrate into normal communities and become contributing and useful members of society.

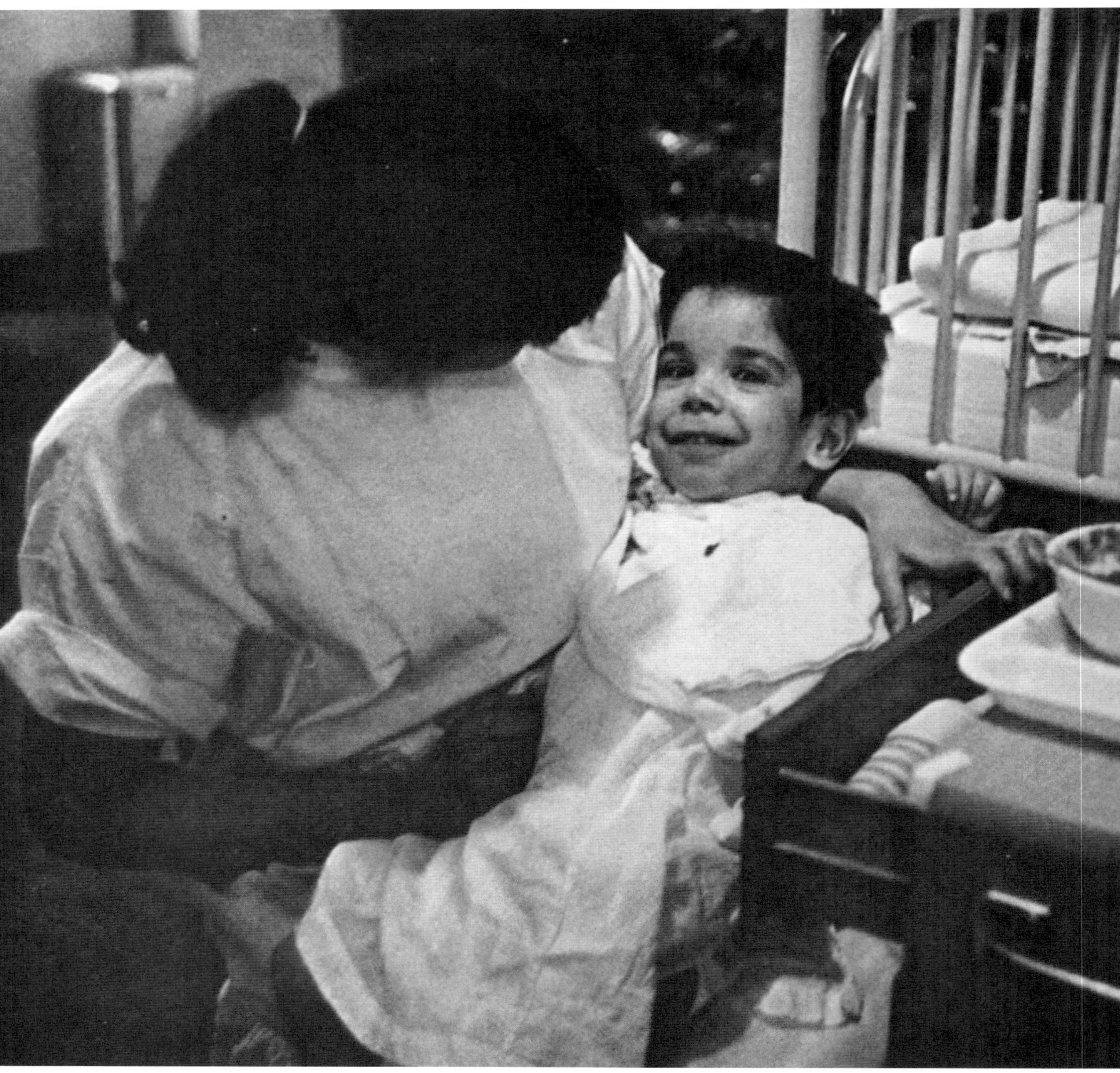

"And had a face like a Blessing."

Miguel de Cervantes

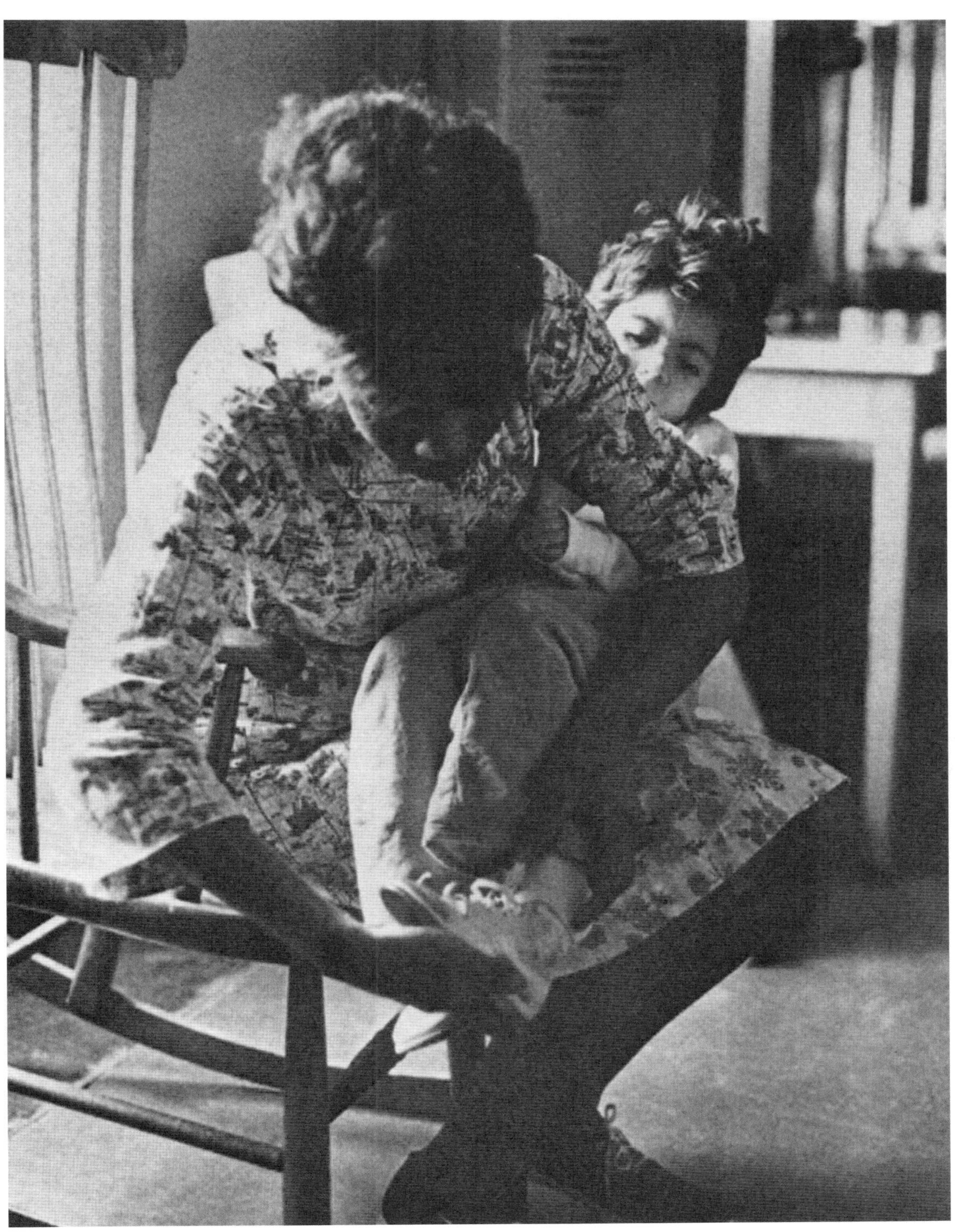

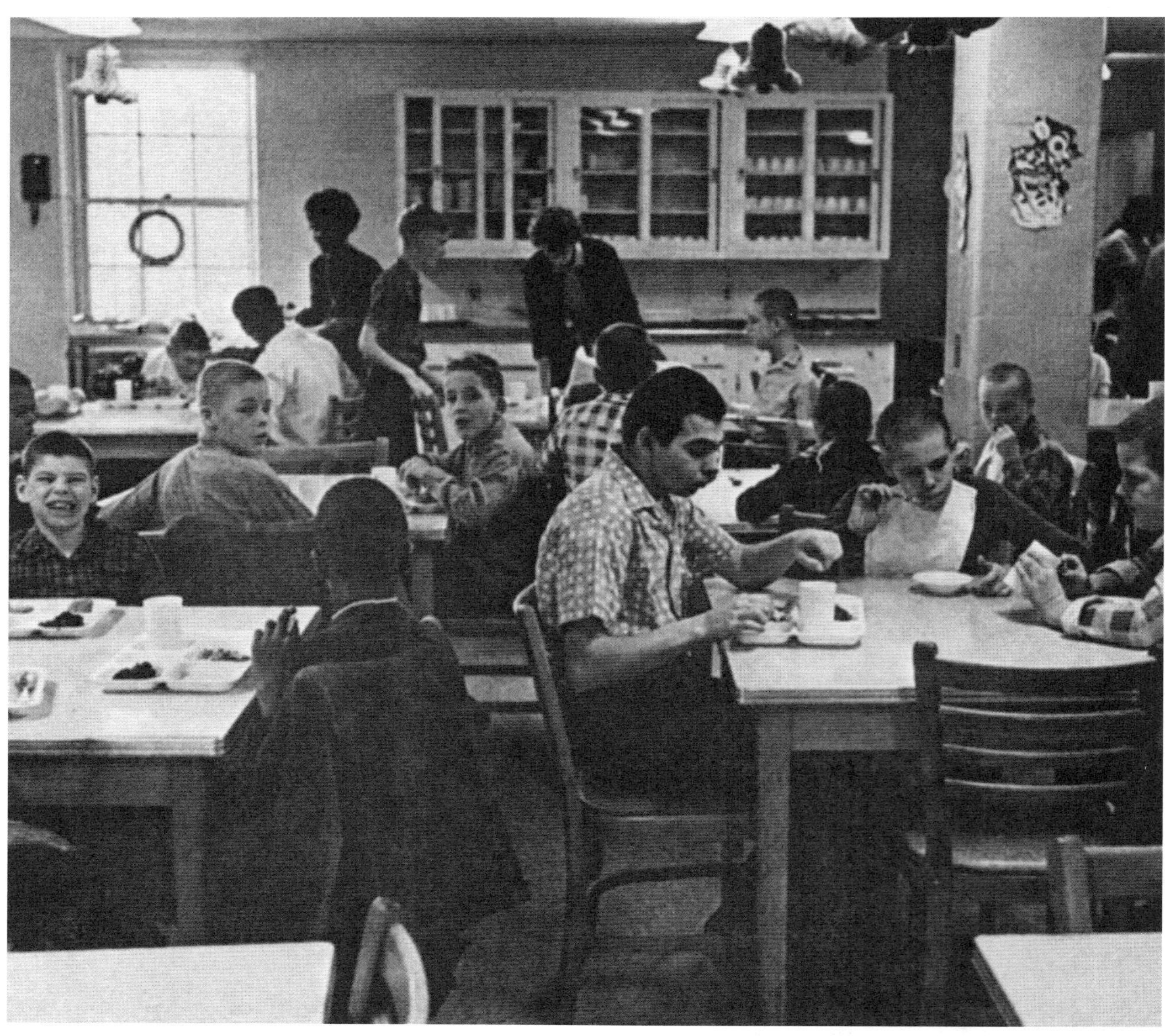

"Youngsters are often not taught to feed themselves; it is easier to drape a sheet around their shoulders and arms and spoonfeed them. They are often not given furniture or toys or help; they might get hurt. The meticulous attention paid to their corporal protection is in sharp contrast to the frequent failure to recognize those important aspects of personal dignity or feeling."

Lewis B. Klebanoff

"Before we start experimenting it would be wise to find out what occurs in the natural situation."

Seymour B. Sarason

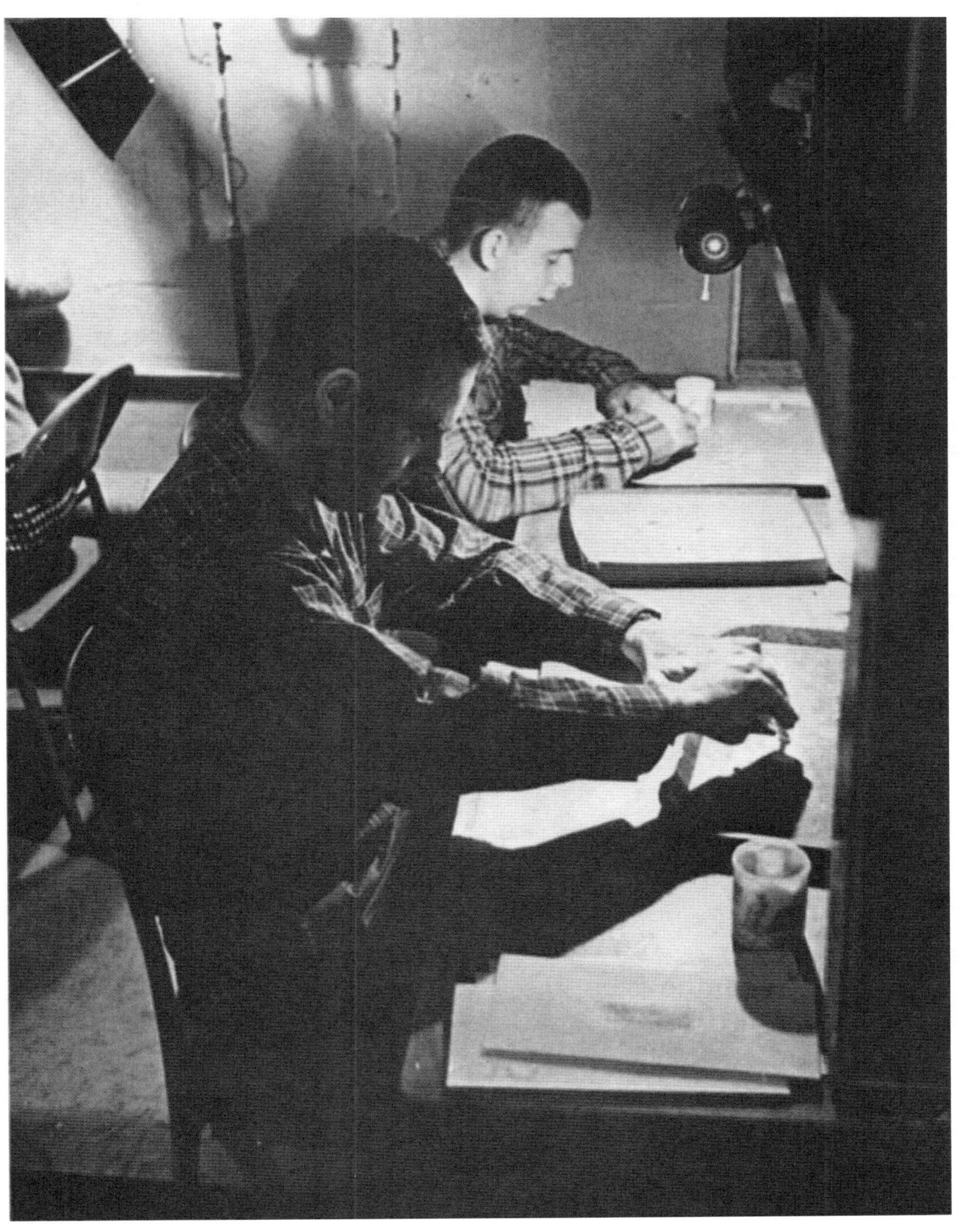

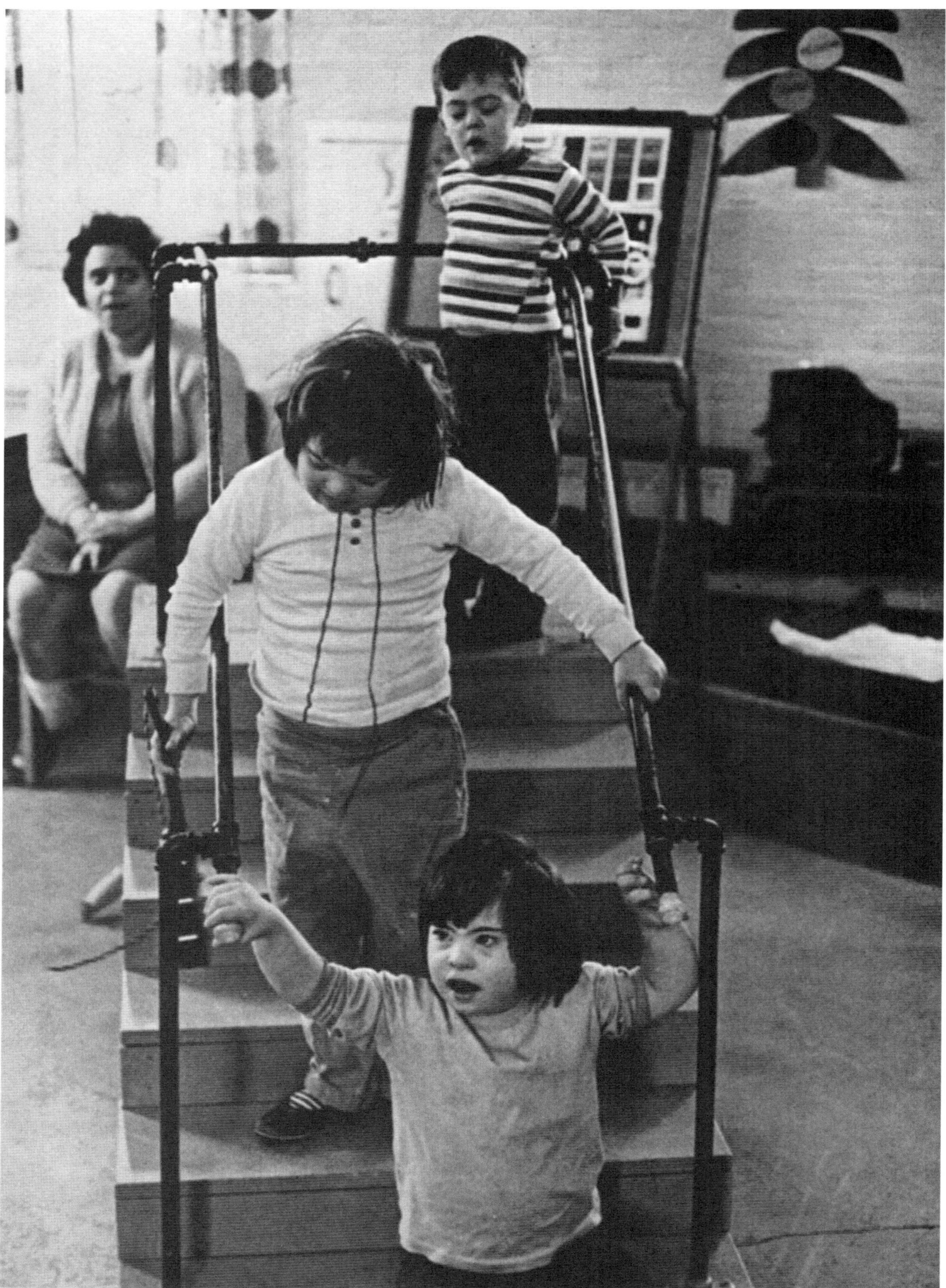

“The greatest discovery of my generation is that human beings can alter their lives by altering their attitudes of mind.”

William James

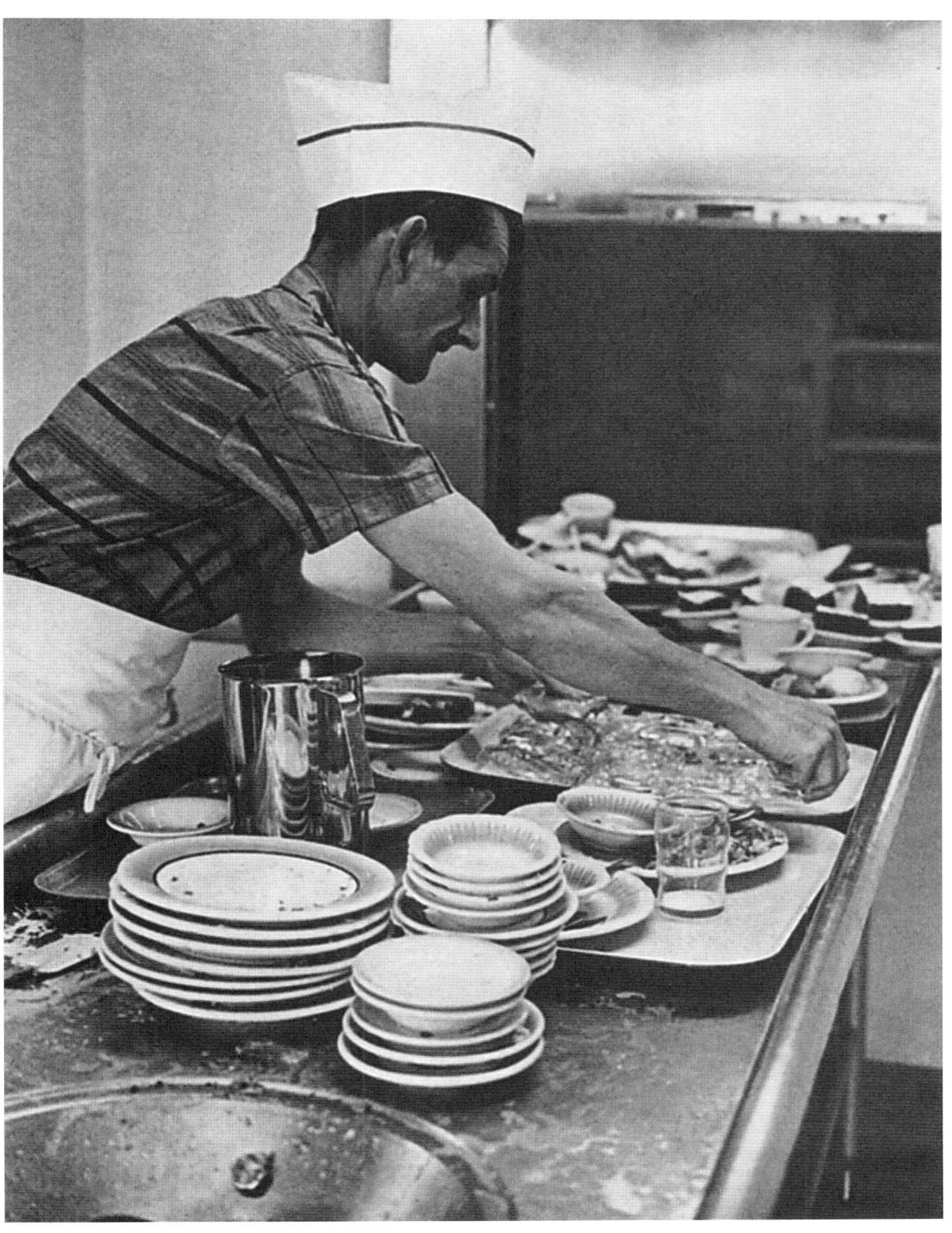

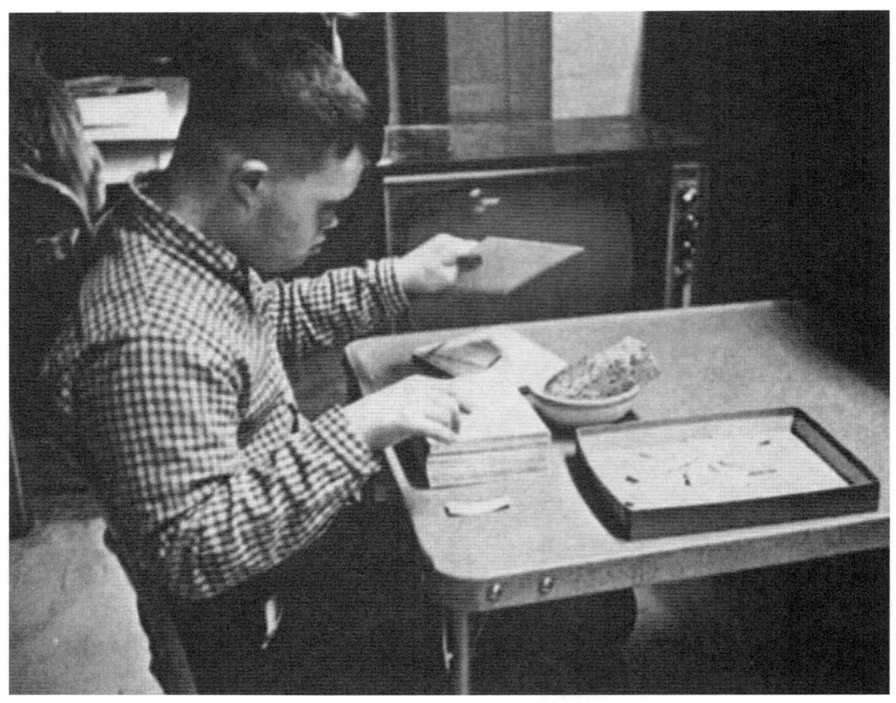

"Genius, that power which dazzles mortal eyes,
Is oft but perseverance in disguise."

Henry Willard Austin

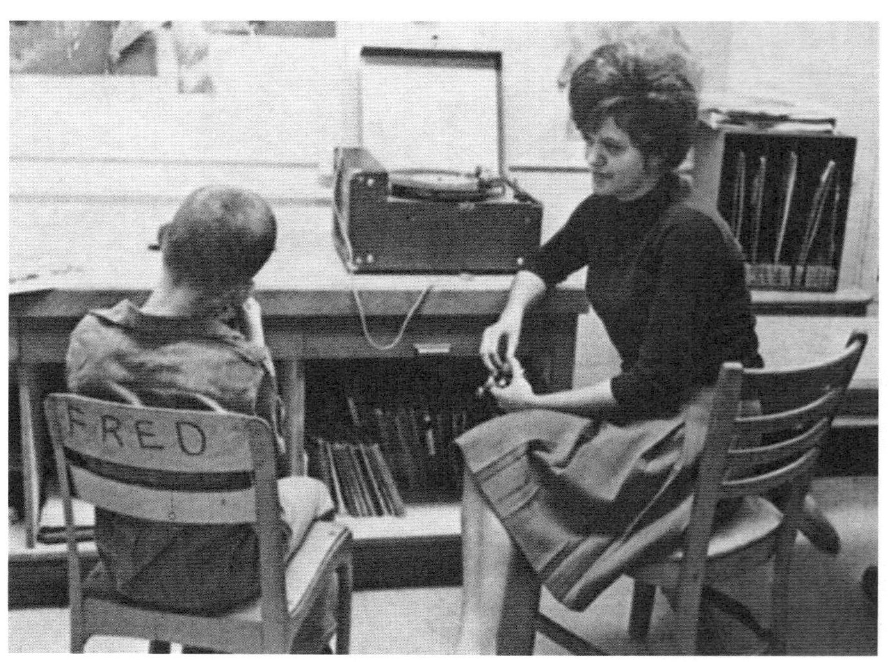



"As with the child, the clinician's most important creation is himself."

Albert T. Murphy

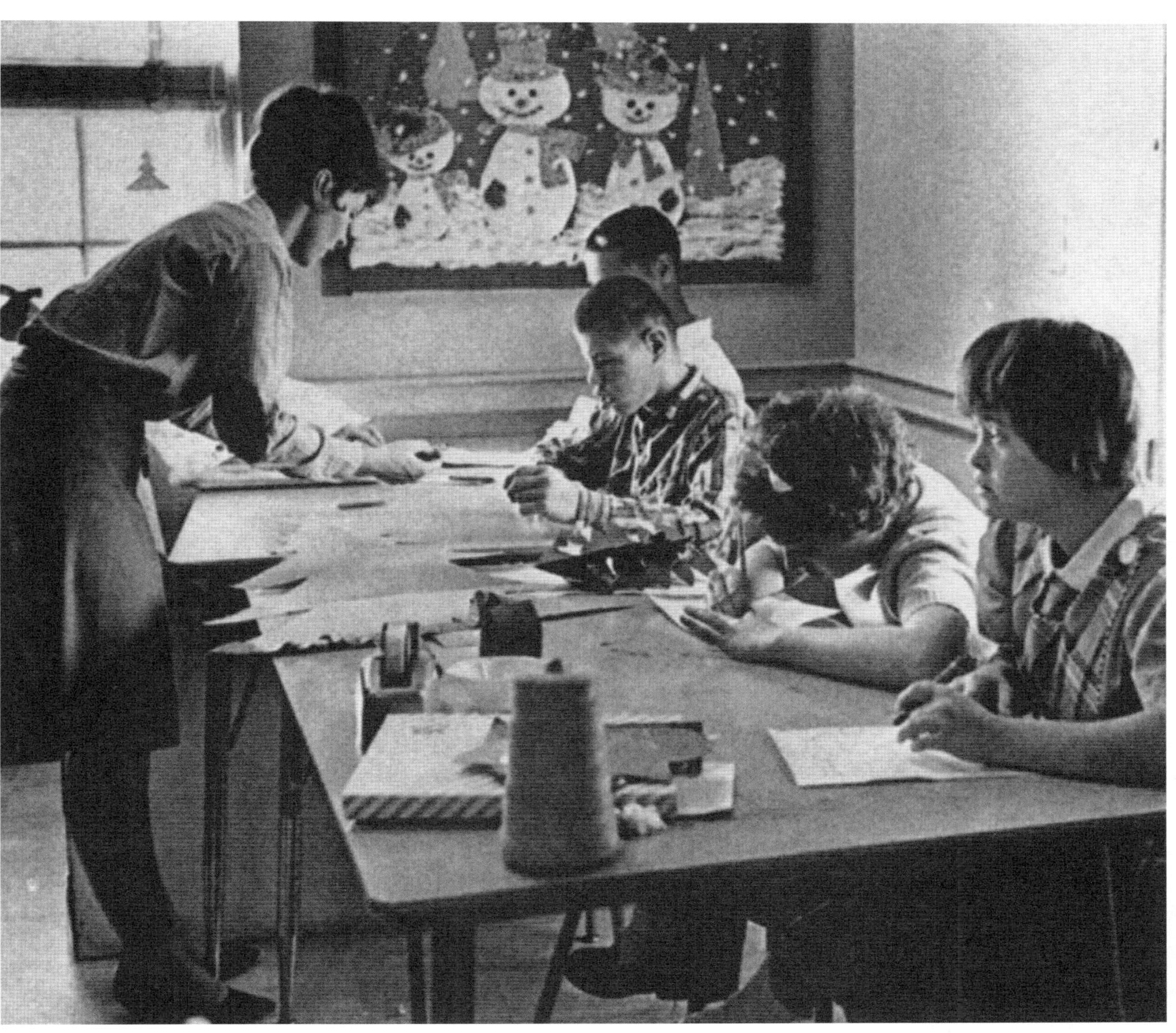

"It is clear that there should be legislation about education and that it should be conducted on the public system. But consideration must be given to the question, What constitutes education and what is the proper way to be educated?"

Aristotle

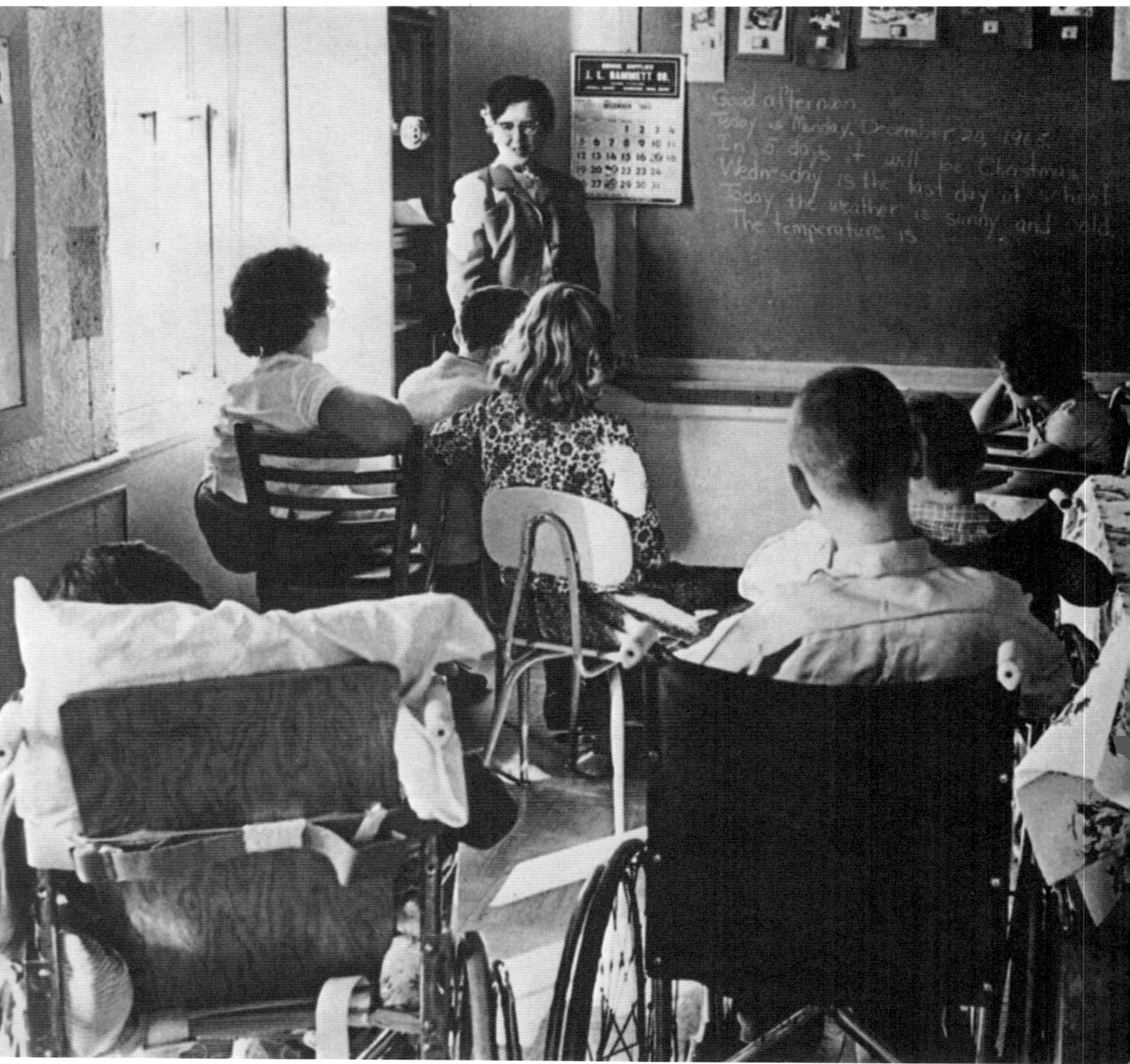

"I was eyes to the blind, and feet was I to the lame."

Job XXIX, 15

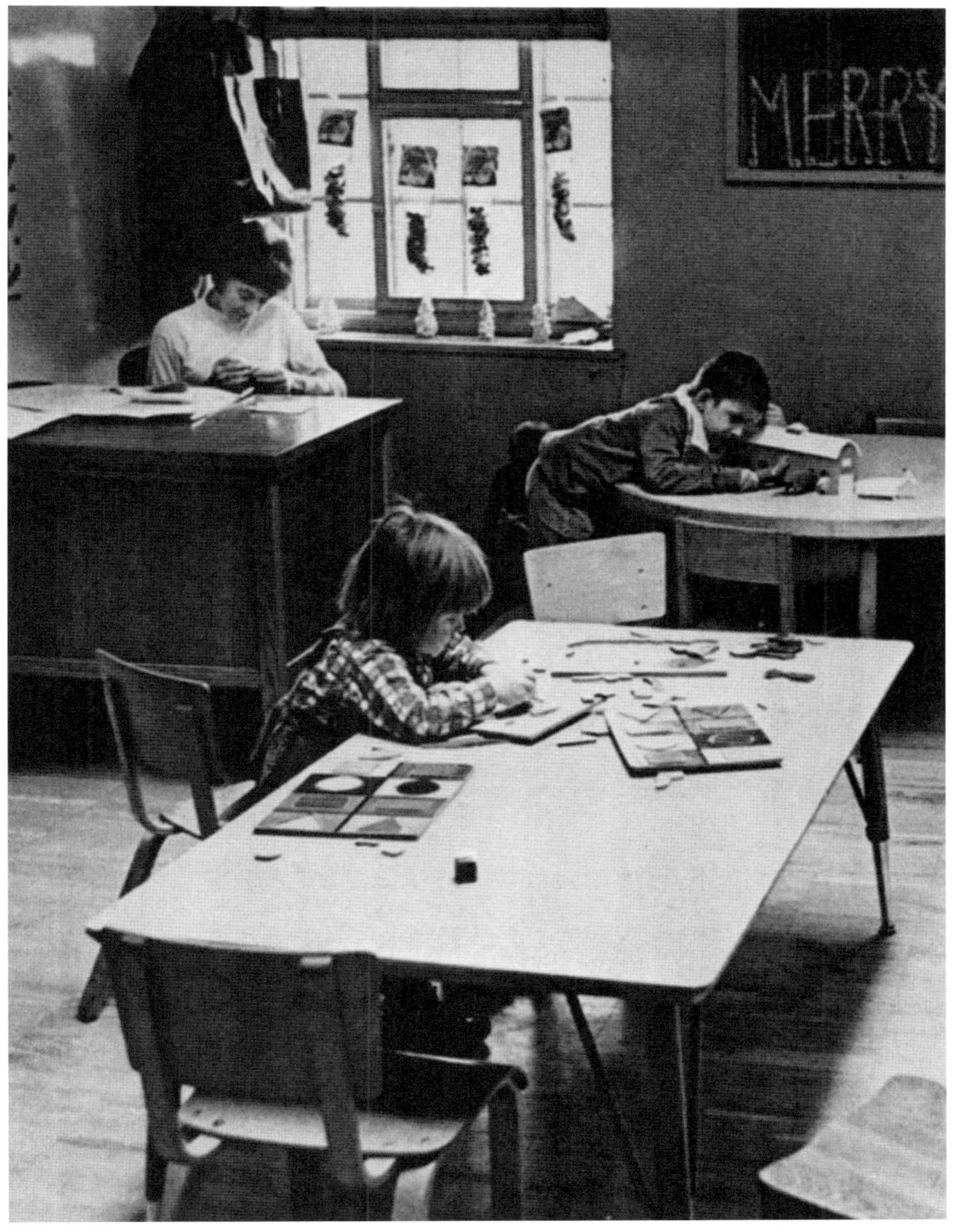

"A teacher who makes little or no allowance for individual difference in the class-room is an individual who makes little or no difference in the lives of his students."

William Arthur Ward

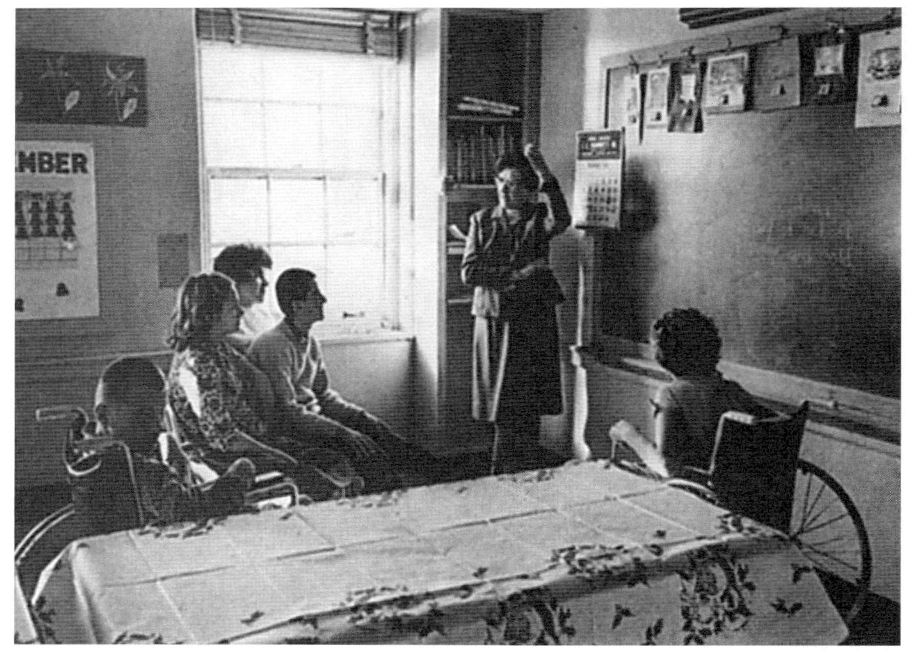

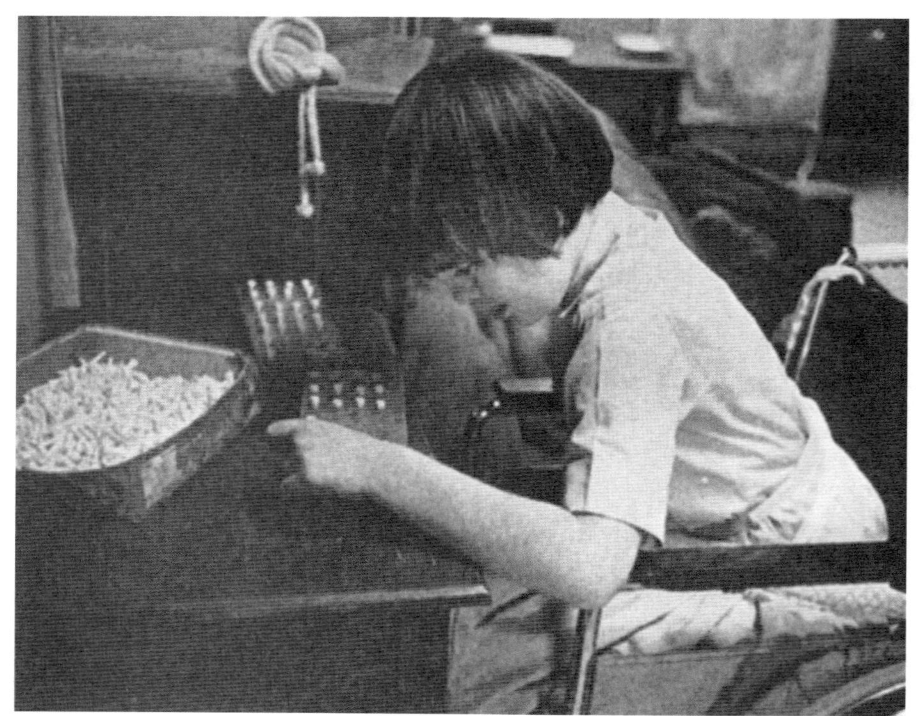

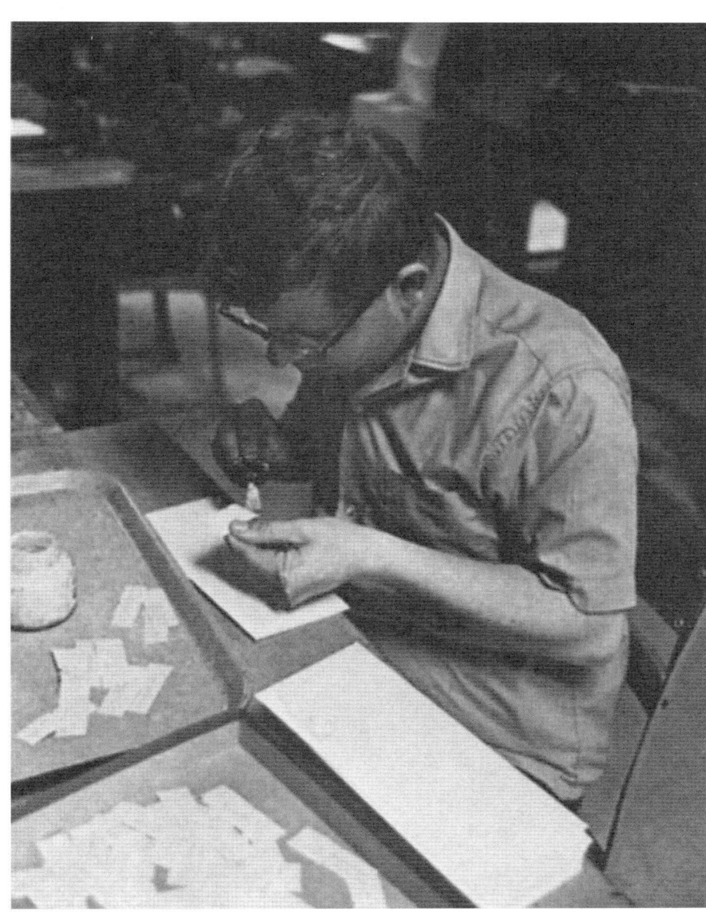

"Love is believing in the fulfillment of another human being."

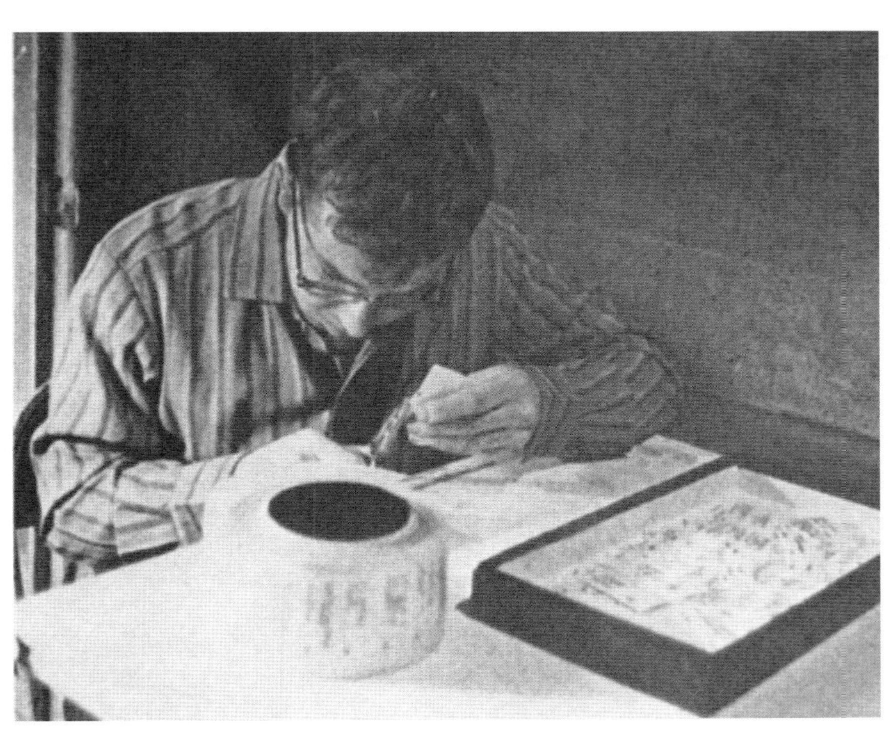

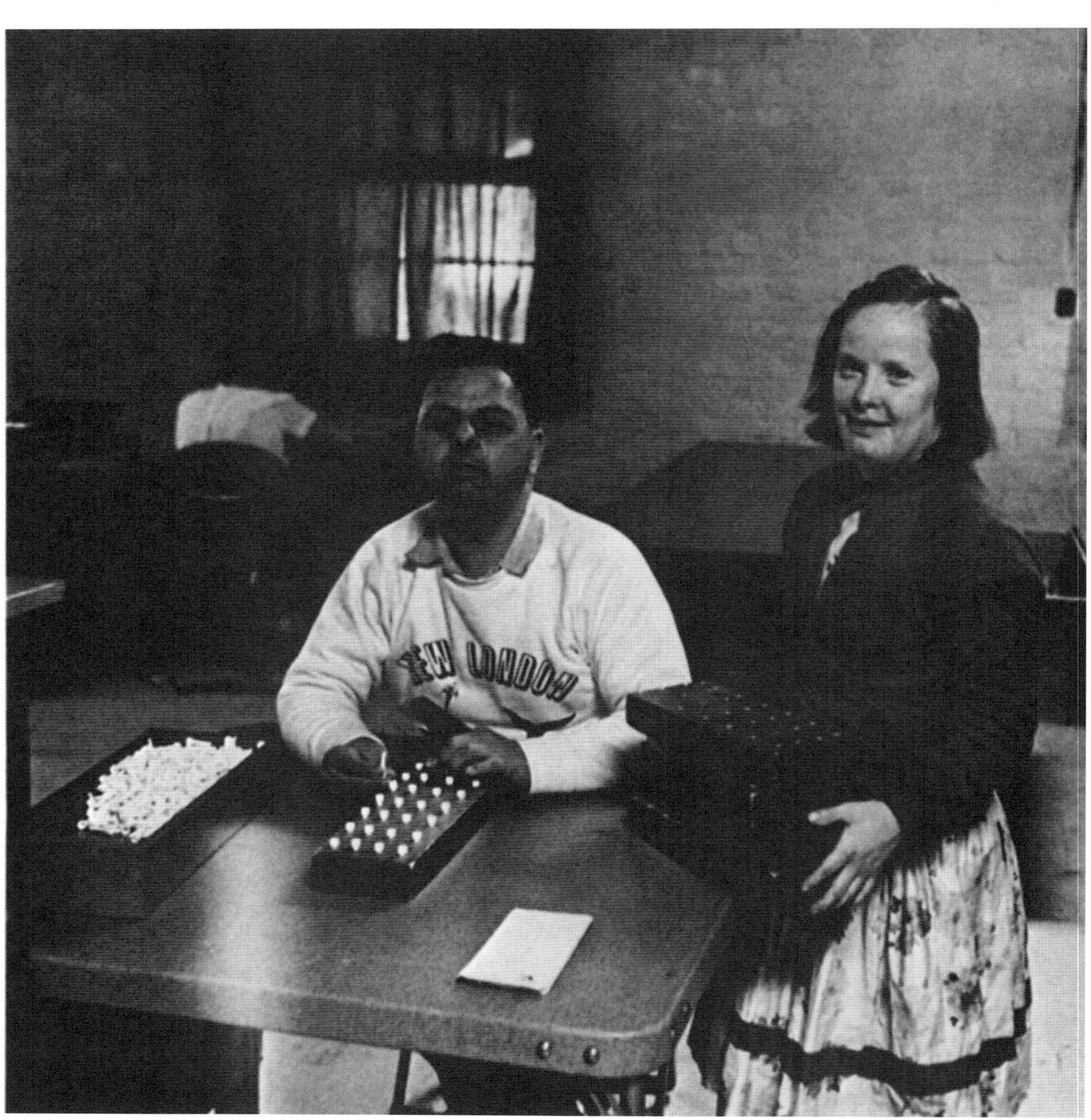

Christmas in Purgatory

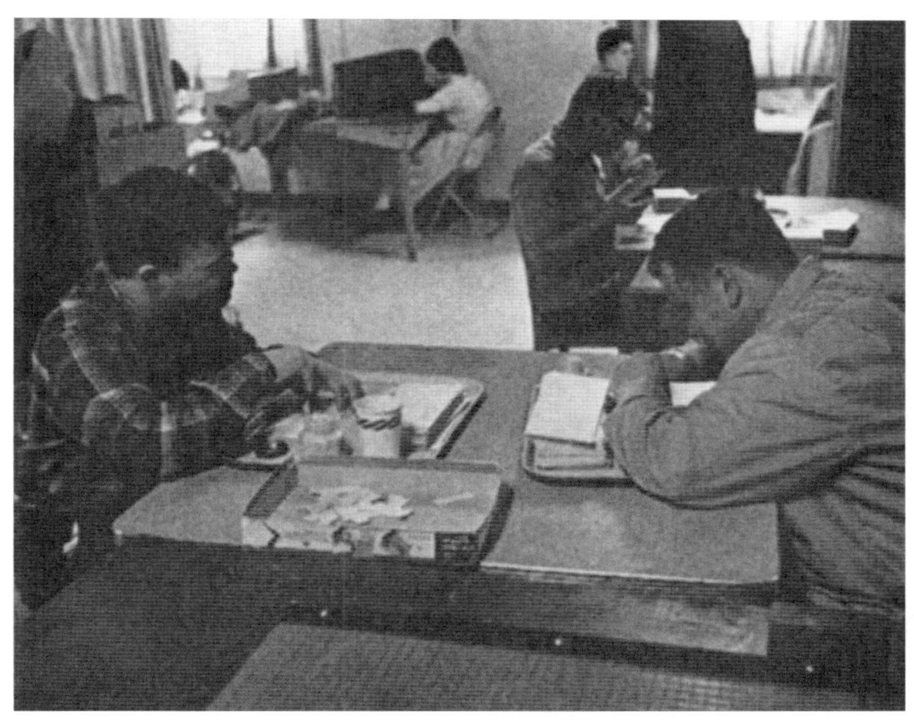

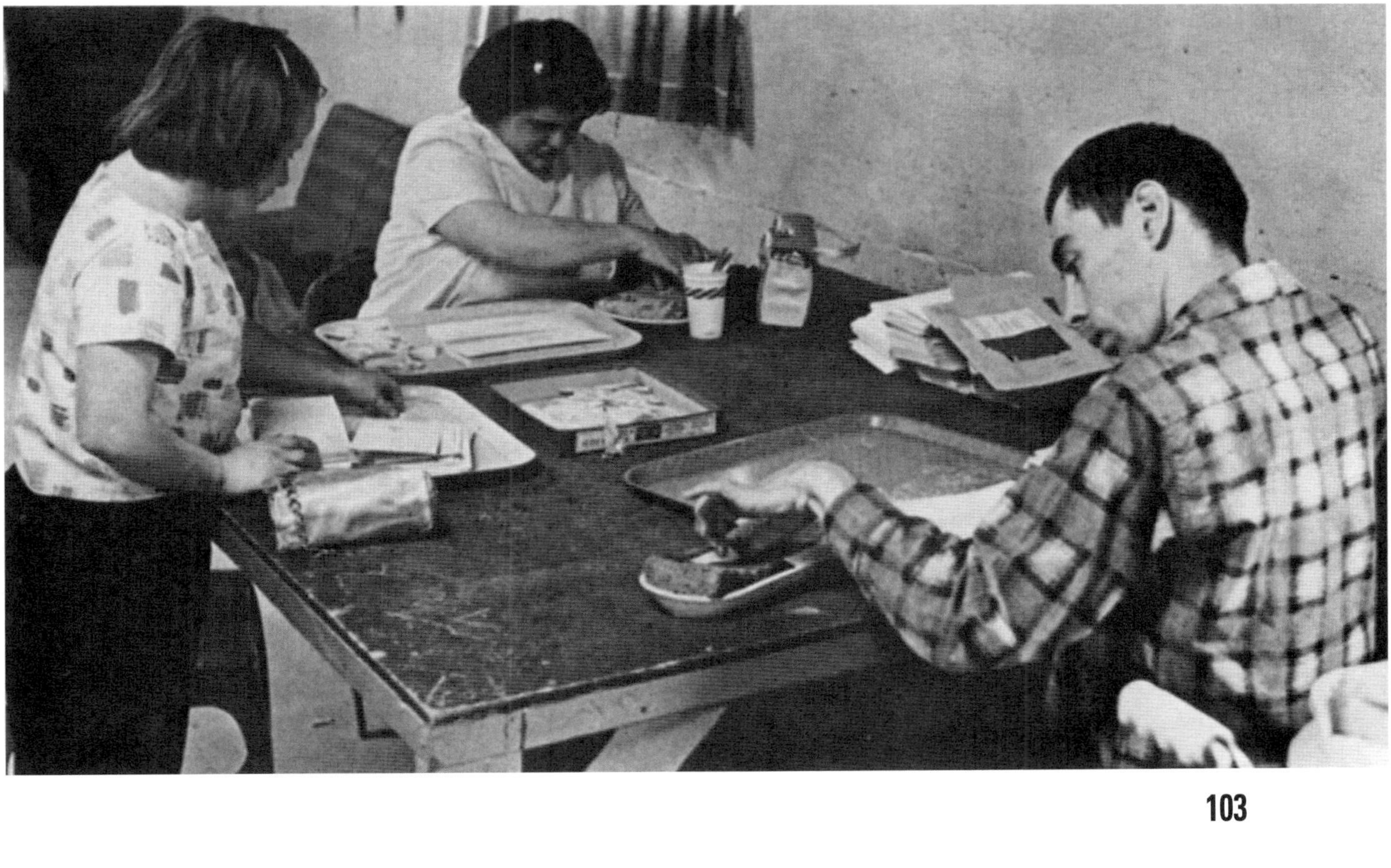

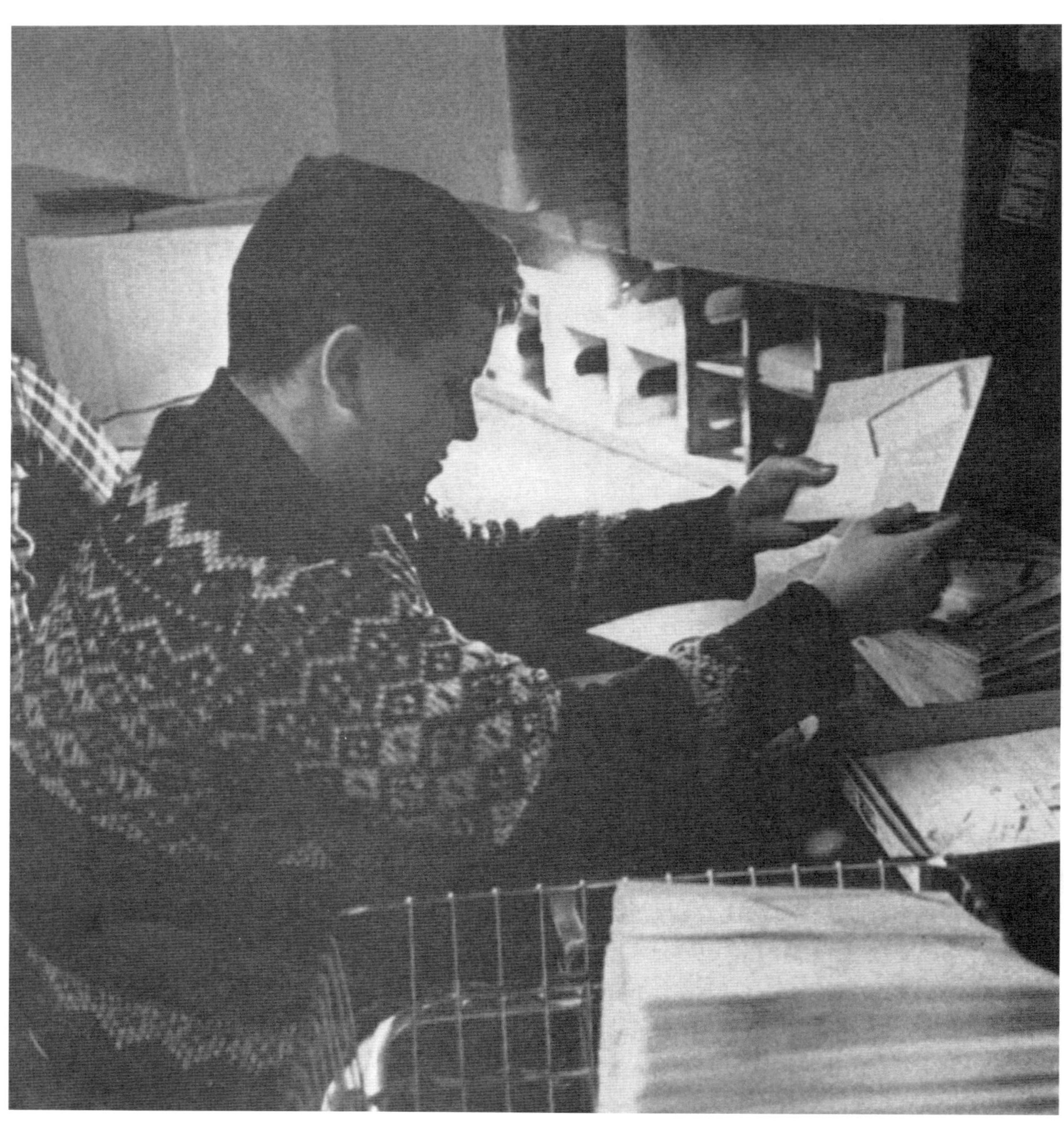

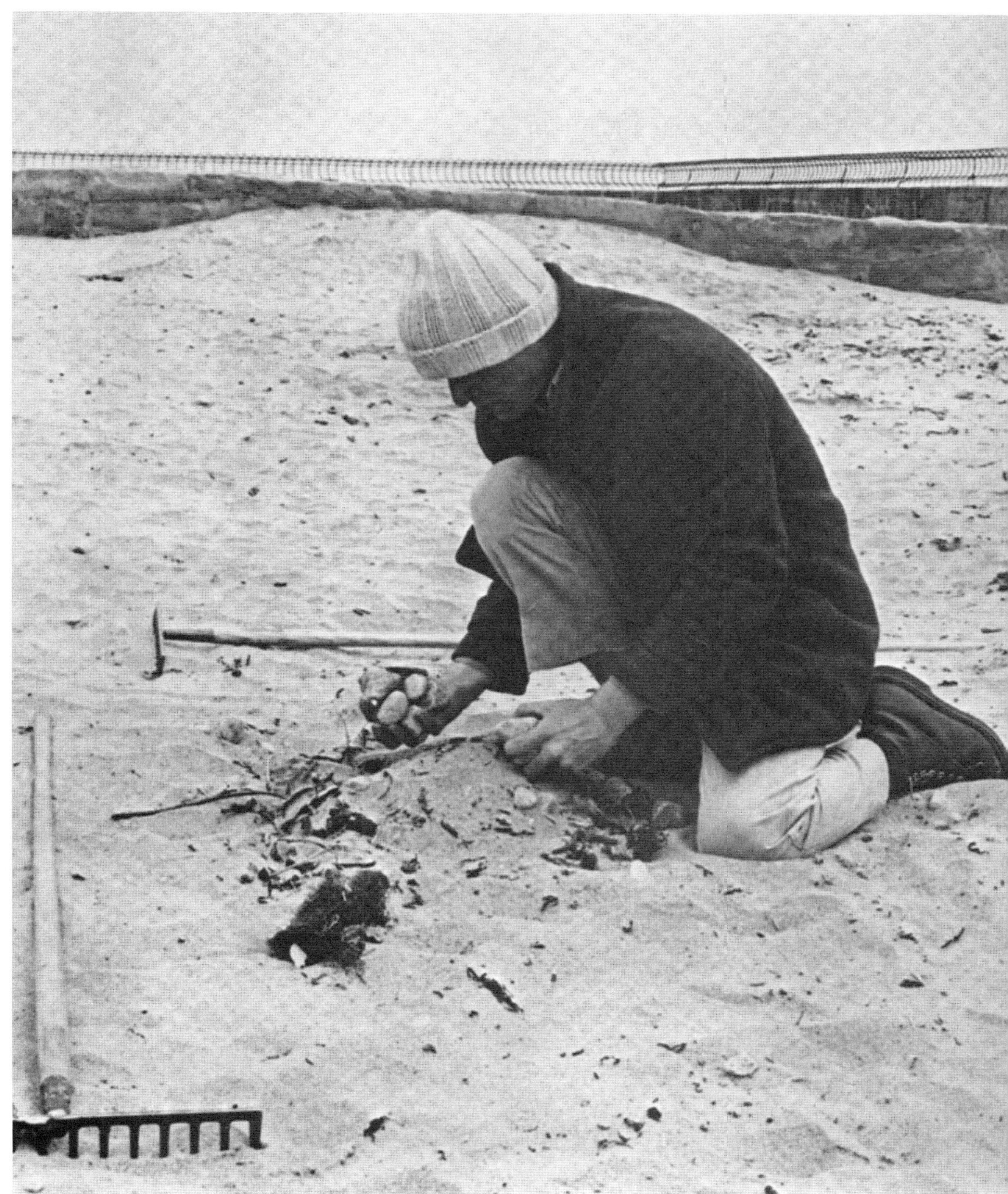

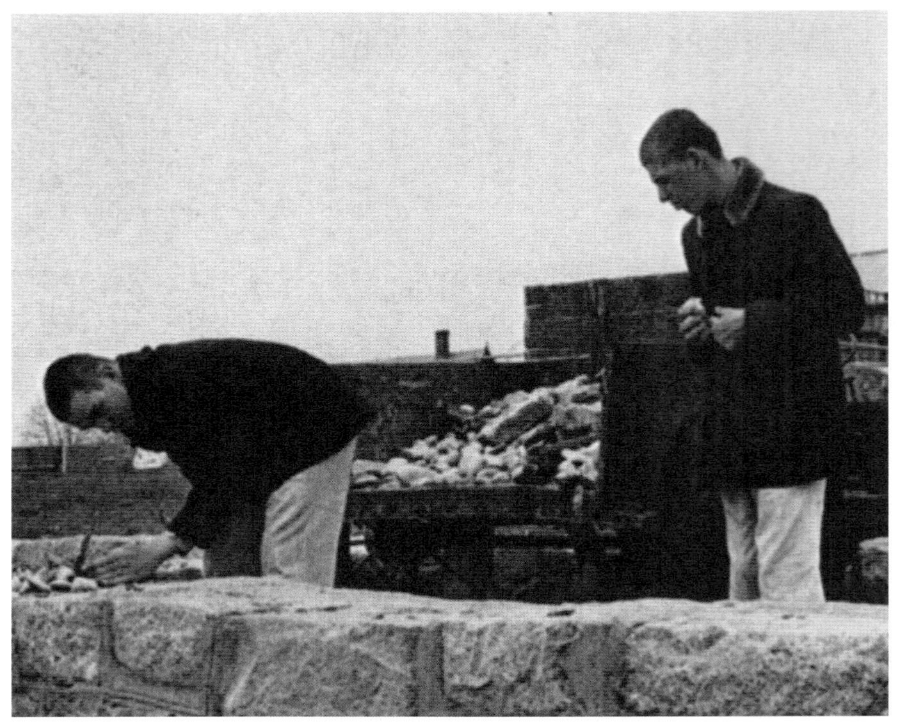

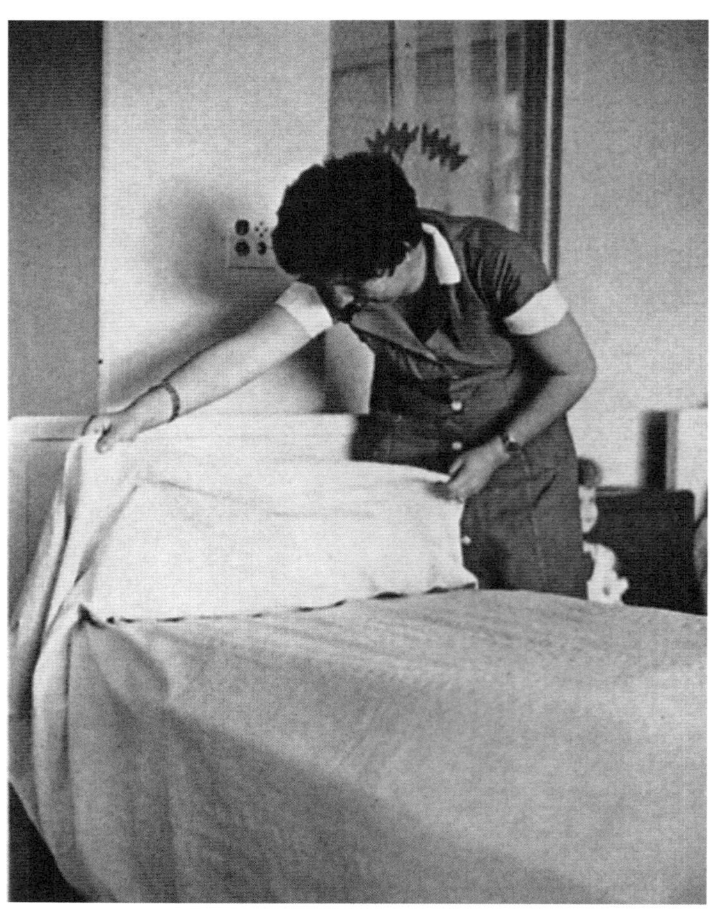

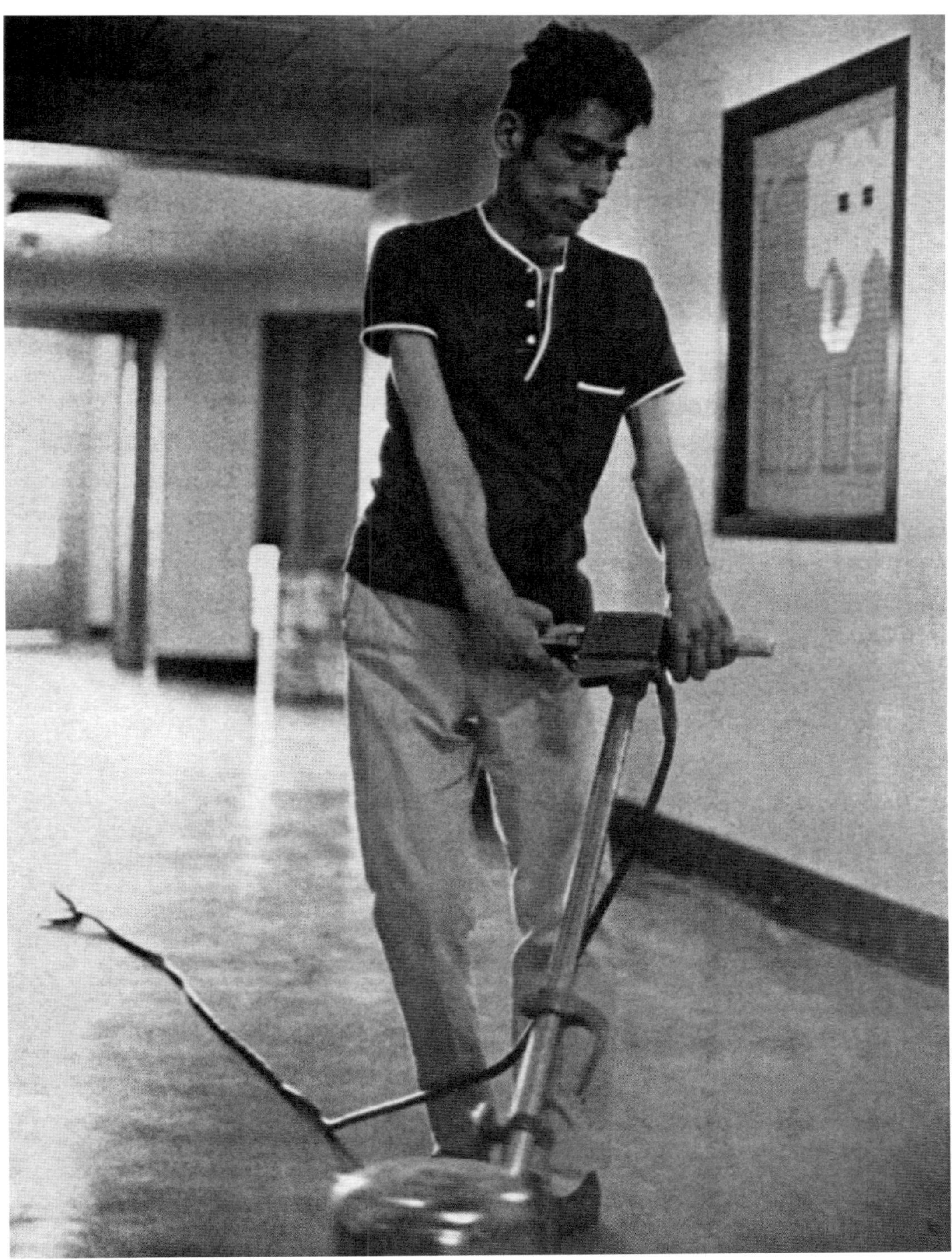

“It could be argued with a good deal of persuasiveness that when one looks over the history of man the most distinguishing characteristic of his development is the degree to which man has underestimated the potentialities of men.”

Seymour B. Sarason

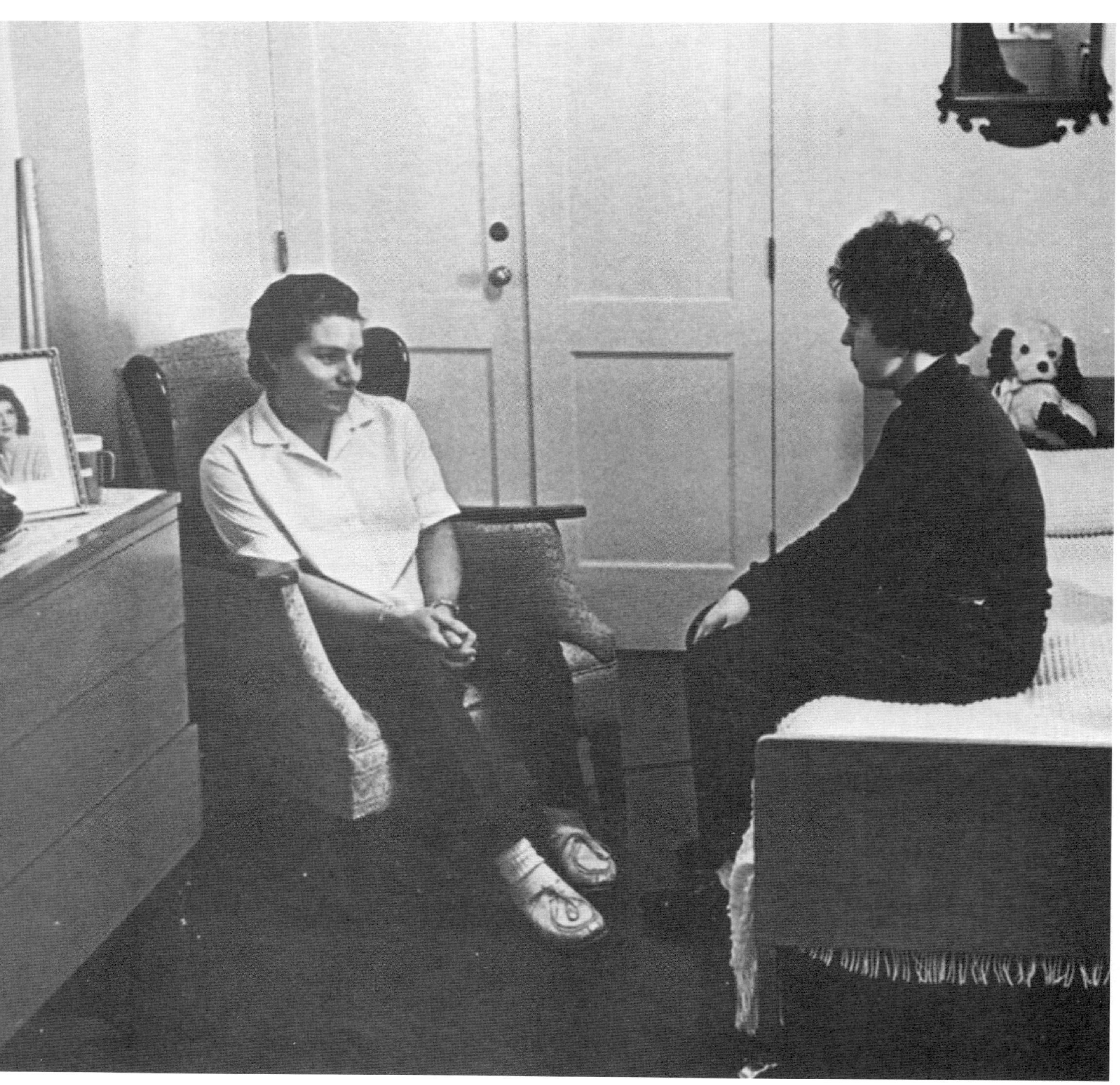

# "Life is a struggle…"

"Life is a struggle, but not a warfare."

John Burroughs

The Seaside is people. It is small. It is expensive to operate, but it isn't expensive as one might expect. The Seaside appropriates approximately twice the amount, per patient, that other institutions do. In contrast with per capita costs in penal institutions, The Seaside has a very modest expenditure. In terms of human suffering—and the potential for human growth—places like The Seaside are among the few really economical government-sponsored facilities of which we know.

There is a shame in America. Countless human beings are suffering needlessly. Countless more families of these unfortunate victims of society's irresponsibility are in anguish for they know, or suspect, the truth. Unwittingly, or unwillingly, they have been forced to institutionalize their loved one into a life of degradation and horror.

We challenge every institution in America to look at itself now. We challenge each institution to examine its programs, its standards, its admission policies, its personnel, its budgets, its philosophy, its objectives. We challenge every institution—and every governor and every legislator—to justify its personnel and their practices, its size and development, and its budget.

Our experiences during Christmas, 1965, require our calling for a national examination of every institution for the mentally retarded in America—an examination that will inspect the deepest recesses of the most obscure back ward in the least progressive state. We call for a national examination of state budgets for the care and treatment of the retarded. We hold each superintendent, each commissioner of mental health, each governor, each thoughtful citizen, responsible for the care and treatment of individuals committed for institutionalization in their state.

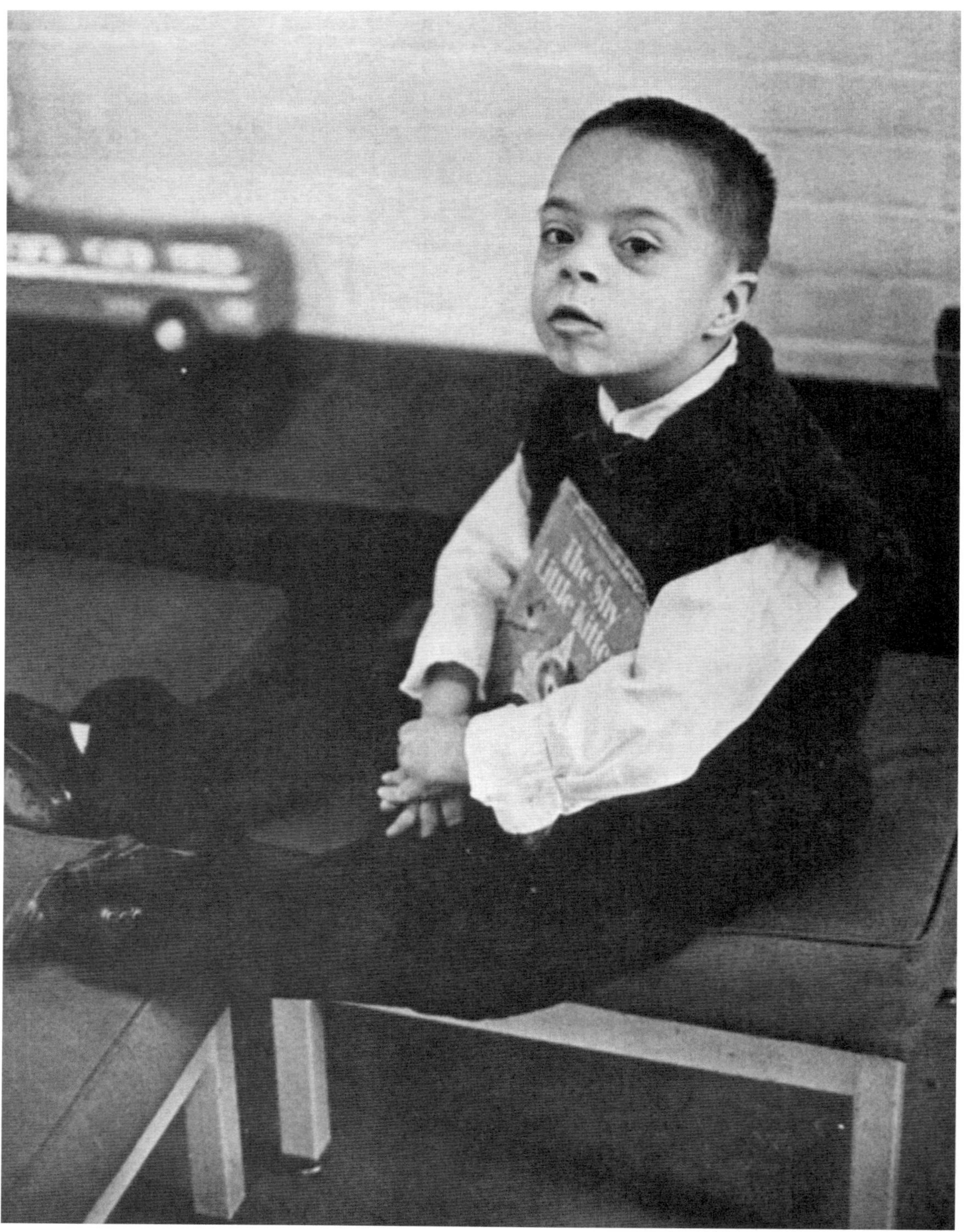

"My most productive moments with subnormal children come about as a consequence of allowing myself to try to experience a childlike sense of wonderment about them as intensely as they approach me with the same attitude."

Albert T. Murphy

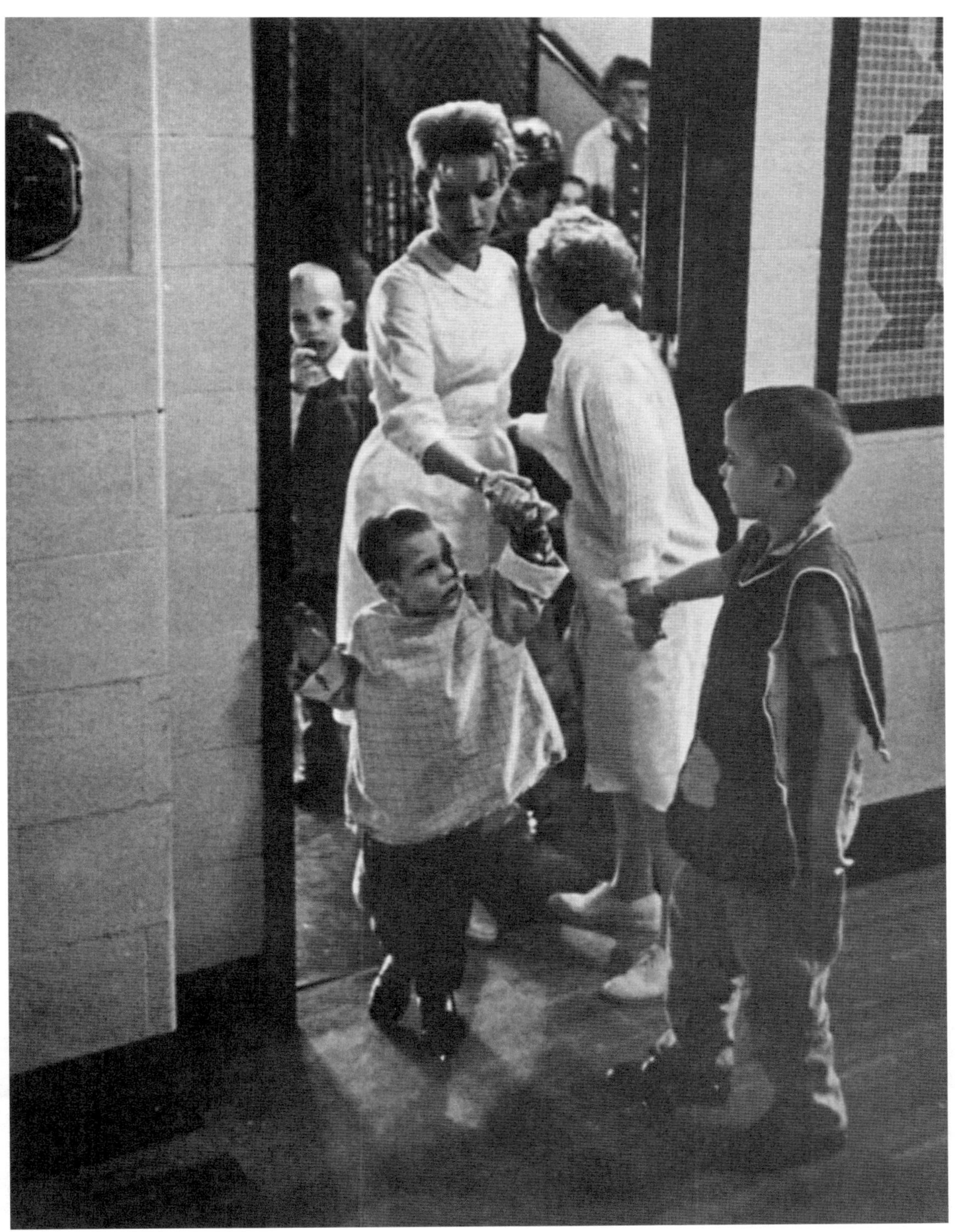

"At each step in history there was always a handful of individuals who saw beyond the man of his time and dreamed of a future when men would be capable of much greater acts in various realms, e.g., the social, moral, and intellectual spheres. Without this handful of individuals it is unpleasant to contemplate how things might have turned out."

Seymour B. Sarason

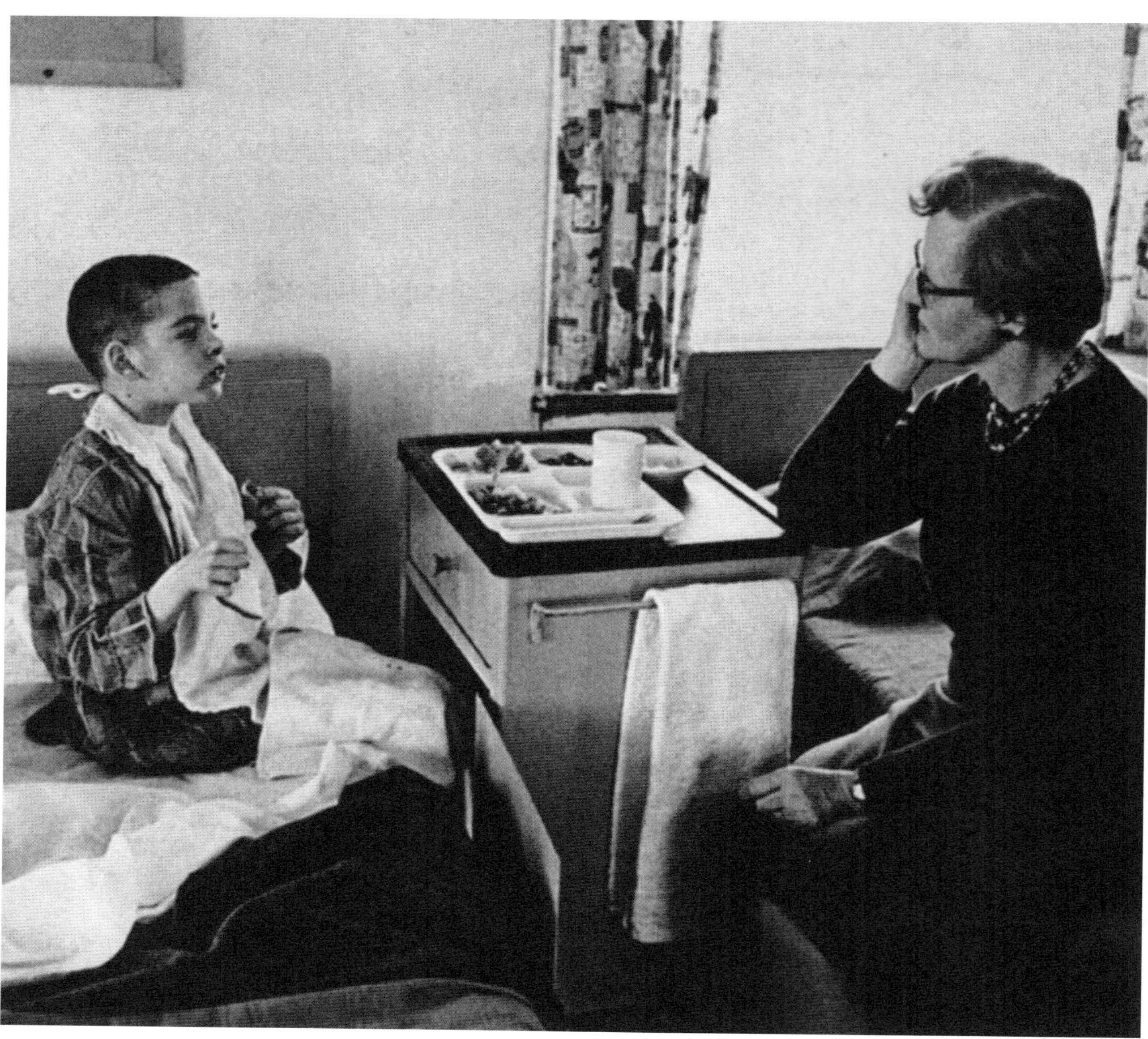

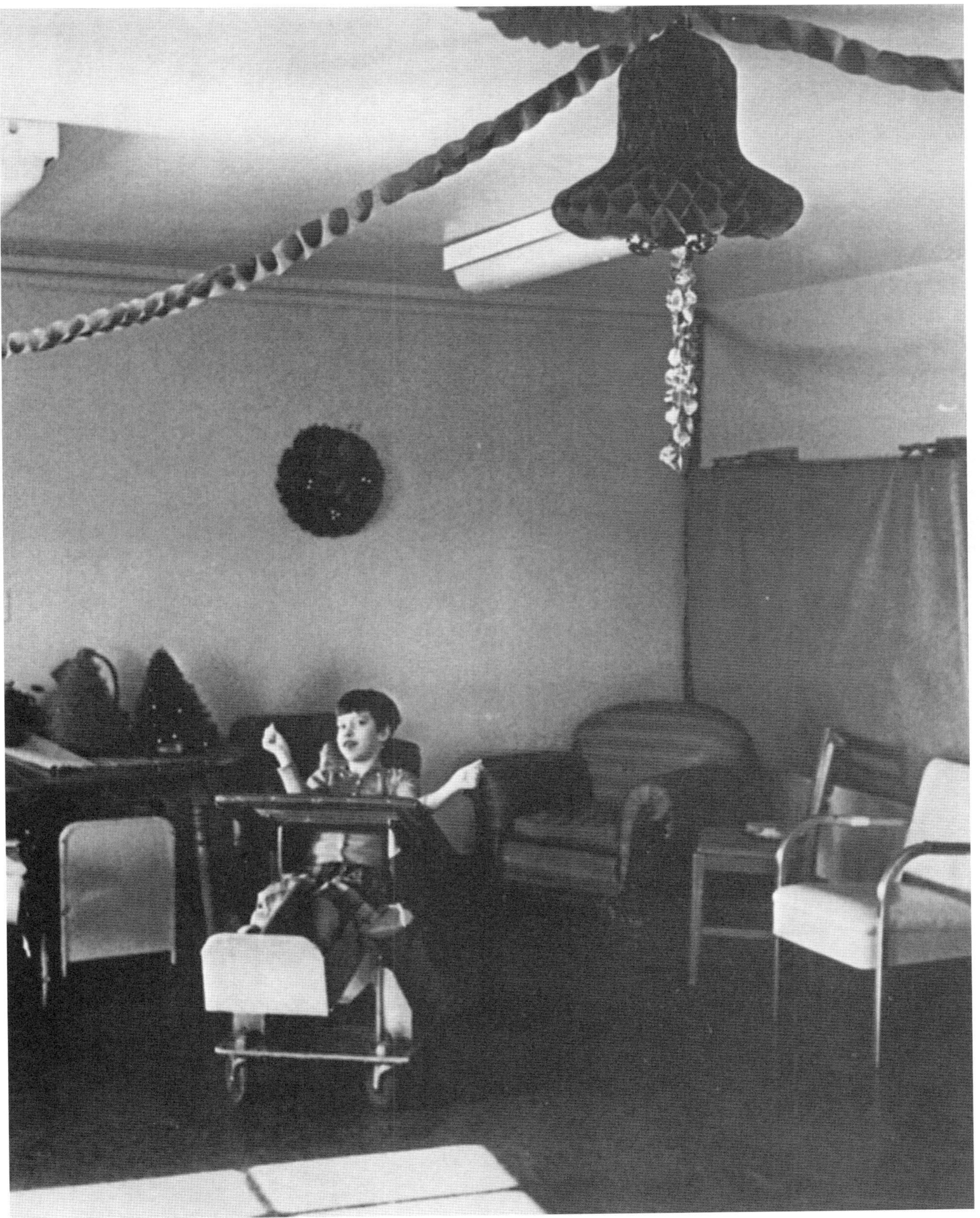

"He who has once been happy is for aye
Out of destruction's reach."

Wilfrid Scawen Blunt

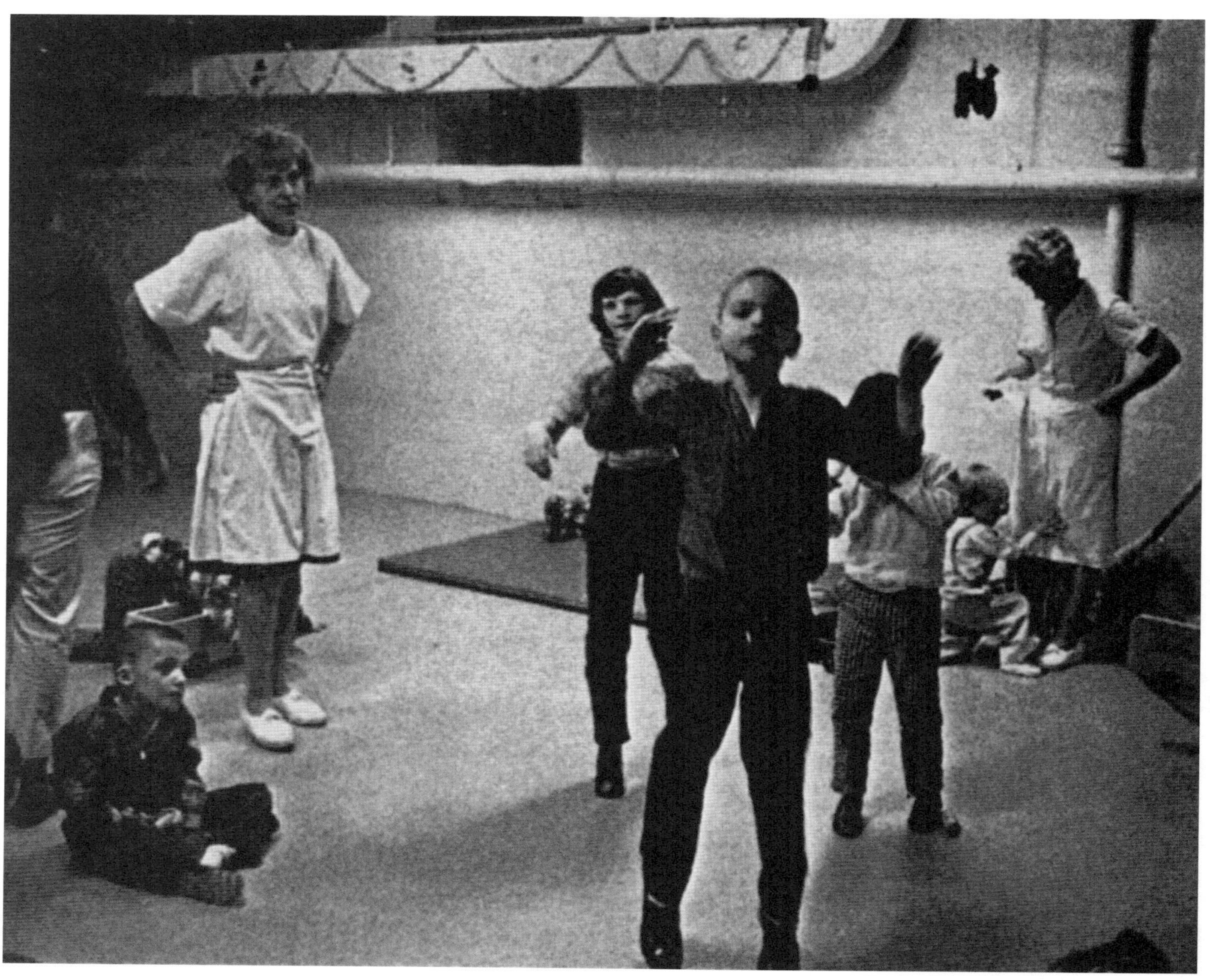

"I believe, like Moses, you can turn the serpent into a rod and learn the lessons which will help you all through life. Remember, unless Moses had handled the serpent he would have had nothing but the bite...there is definitely a place for you and the Design for all of us holds nothing but good."

Margaret A. Neuber

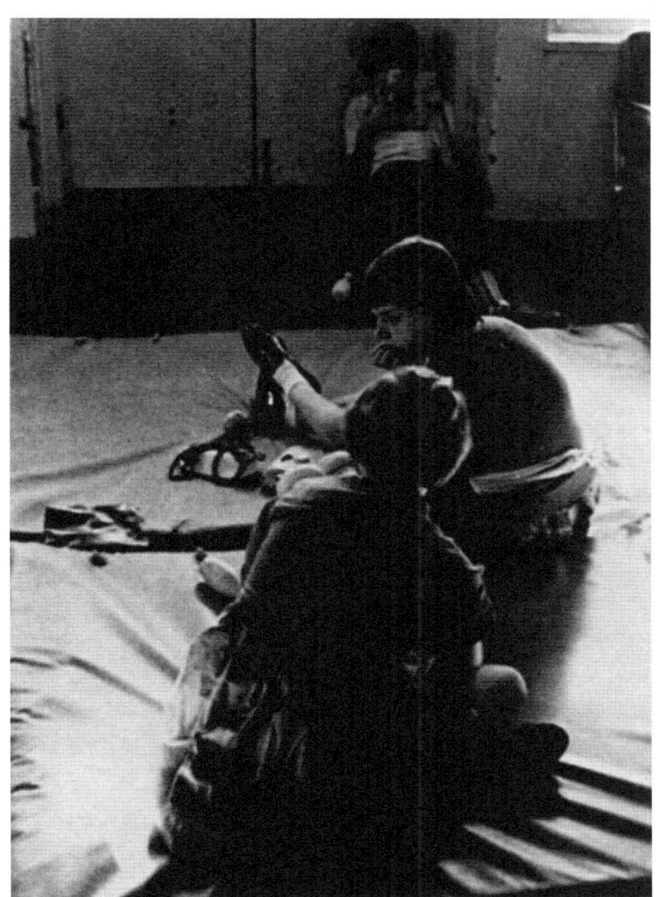

"There's a time for some things, and a time for all things; a time for great things, and a time for small things."

Miguel de Cervantes

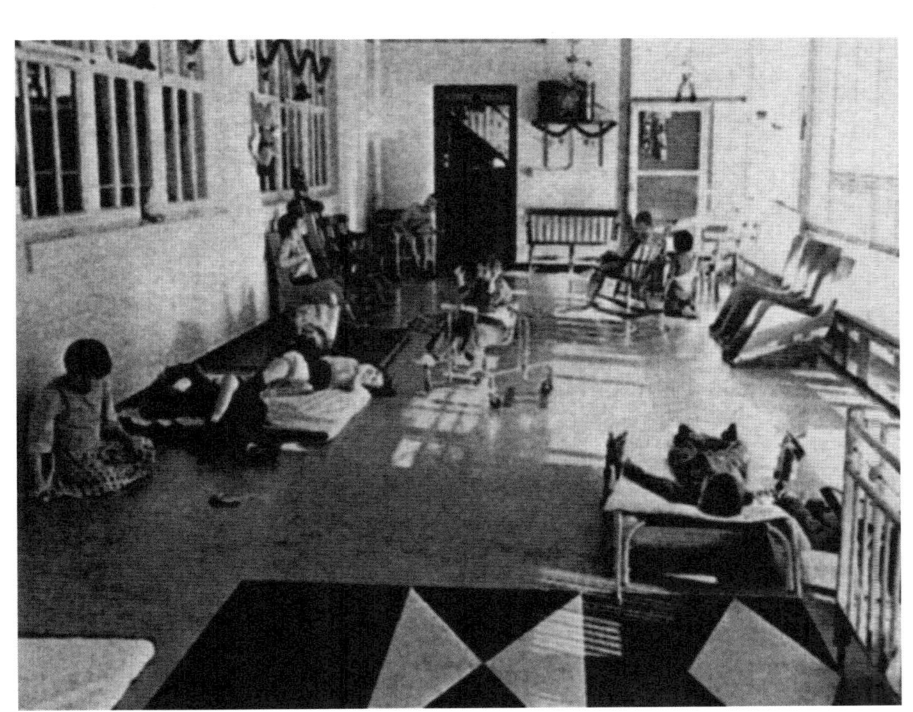

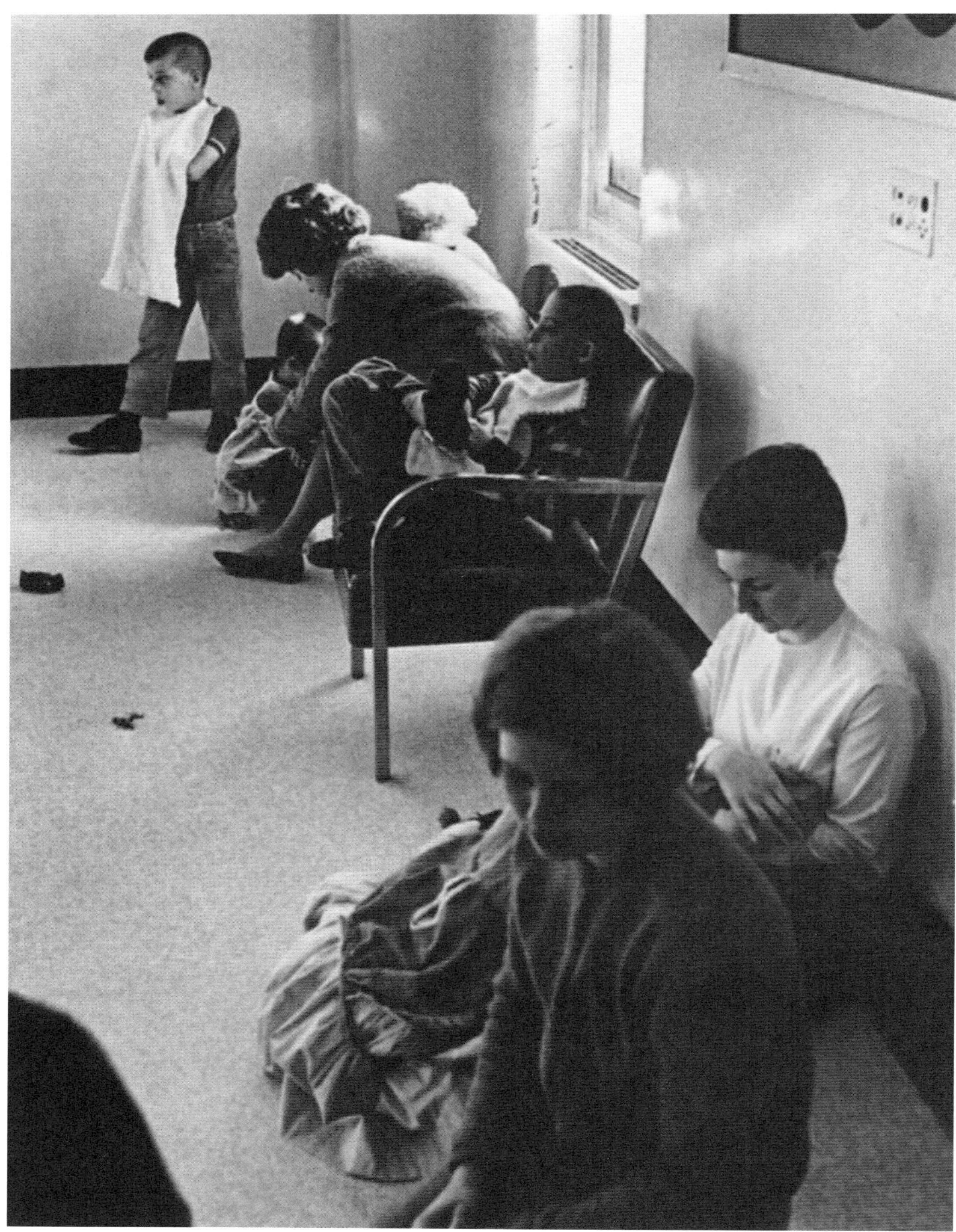

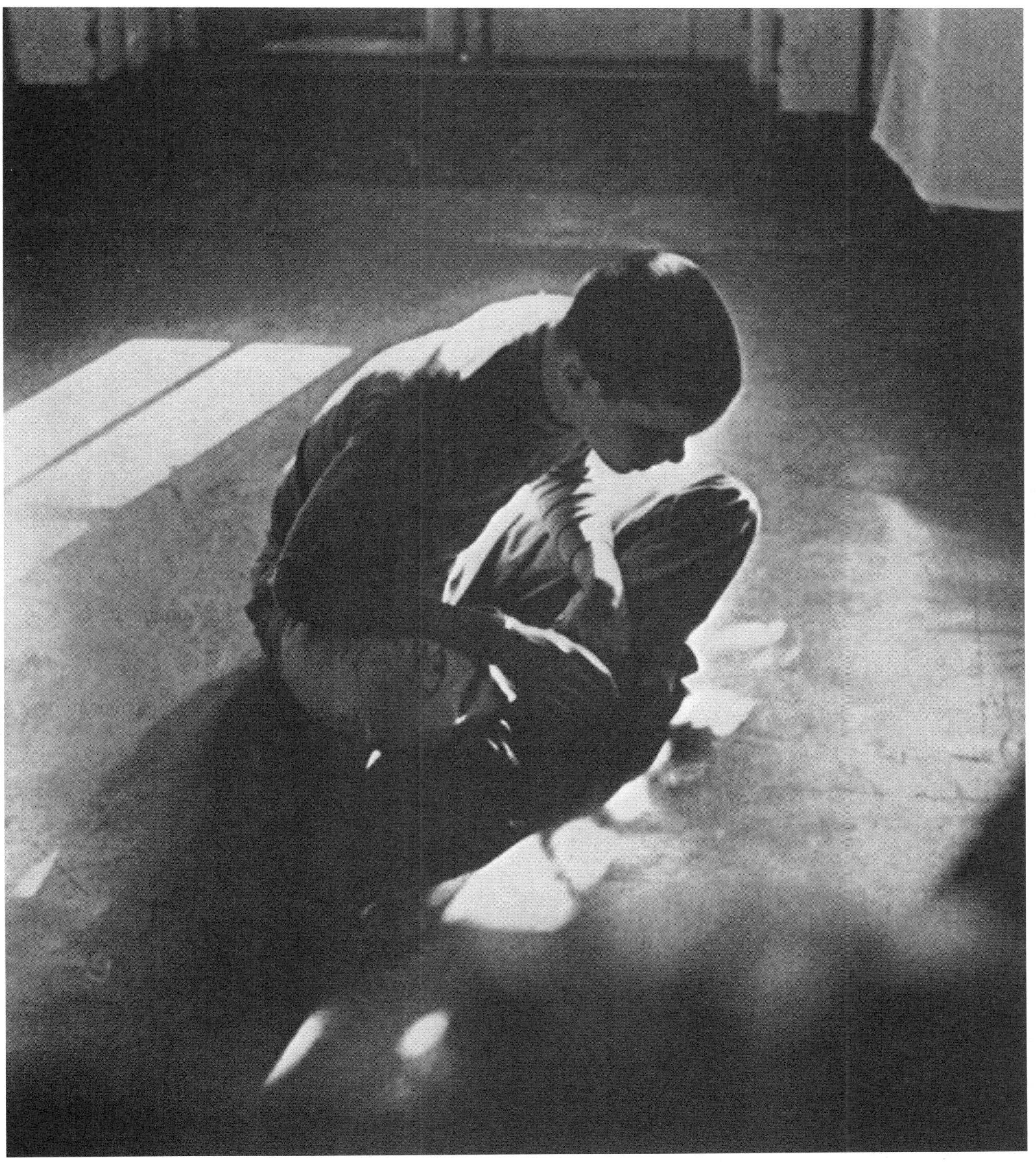

"There is nothing inherent in disability to produce handicap. It is not for behavioral science to find out whether or not this is true, but to make it become true."

Frank Garfunkel

117

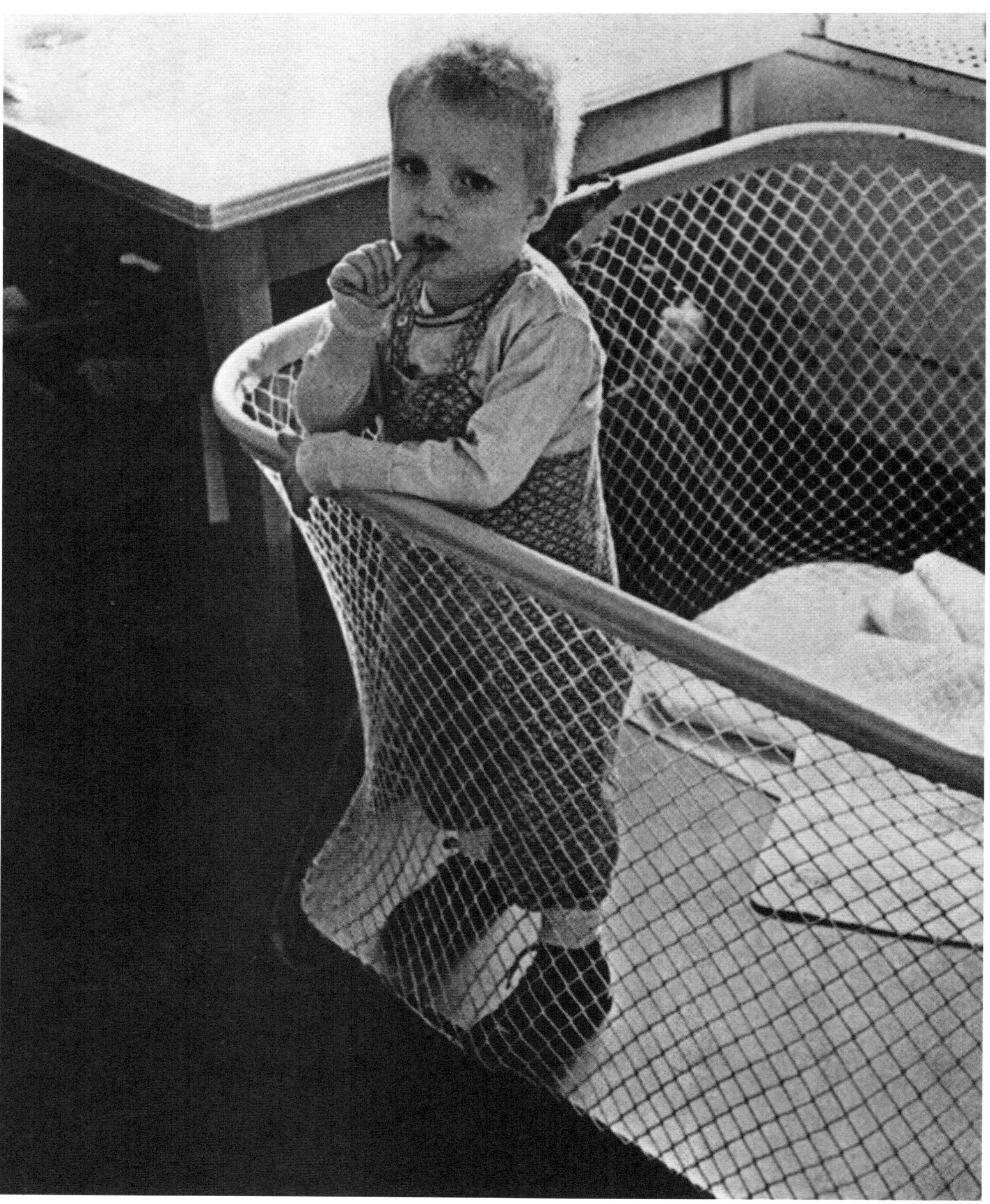

"It is within man's province to educate his intelligence. However, this goal will not be achieved without a great deal of sustaining and integrated research."

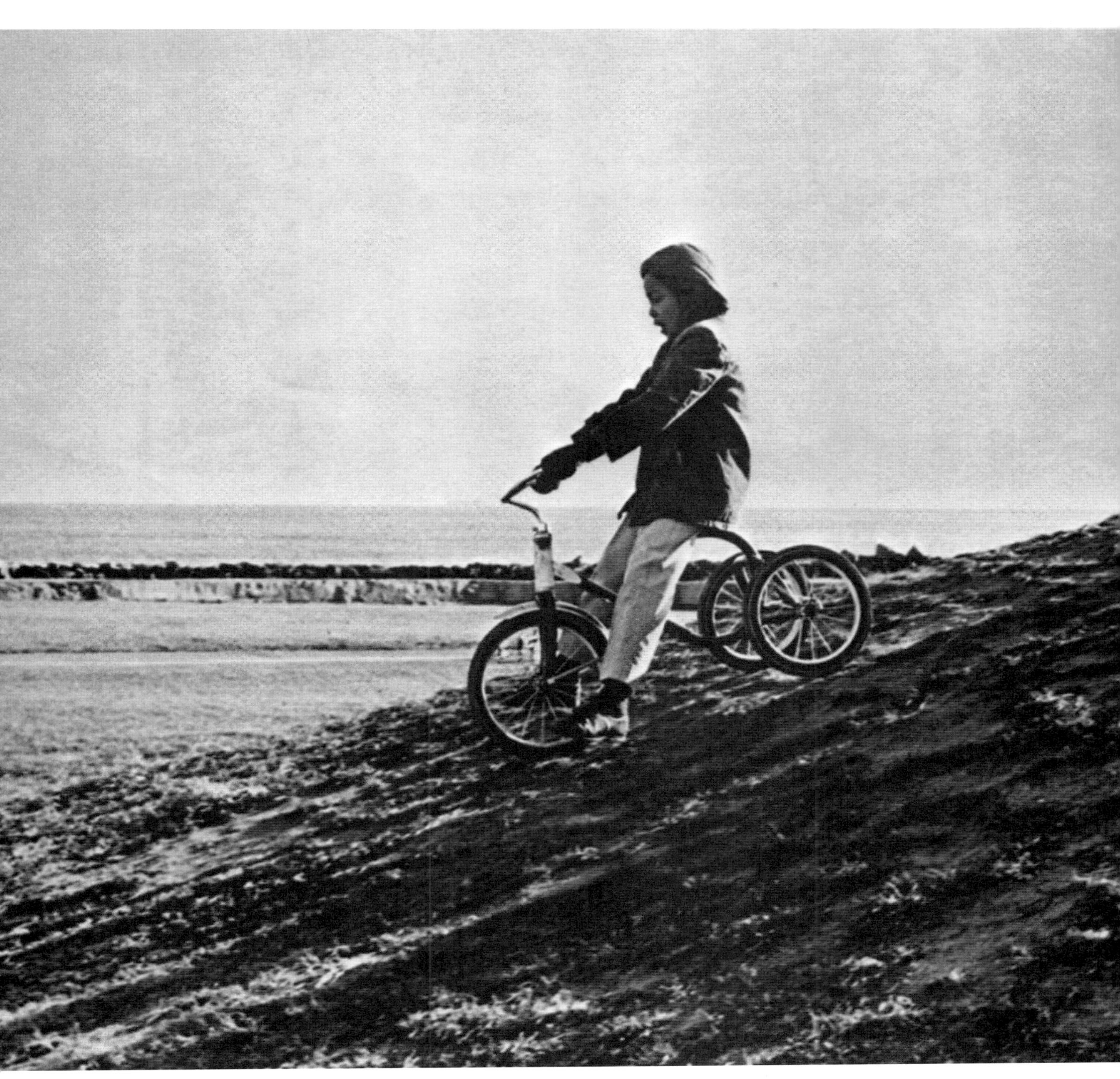

# AFTERTHOUGHTS

<blockquote>

"The triumph of evil requires
only that good men do nothing."

</blockquote>

Since we have visited the institutions described in this book, we have shown and discussed our story with a heterogeneous but carefully selected number of people. Their backgrounds range from those in very high public office to undergraduate college students preparing to be special class teachers. Editors of two of the largest and most influential news magazines previewed and discussed this book with us.

Popular opinions convinced us that this story must be brought to the American people as soon as possible. In discussing this work with so many very knowledgeable persons, we were able to resolve some of our anxieties about the possible adverse reaction to the publication of this study. Further, we were able to conceptualize a plan to correct those conditions we observed.

The major questions that dictated caution and deliberation before a thoughtful answer could be found were concerned with whether or not our work represented an invasion of privacy of certain individuals, on the one hand, and that the general public has a right to be protected from the knowledge of degradation, on the other. As far as invasion of privacy is concerned, we have learned that—from a legal point of view—this is a very ambiguous matter. Although we were forced to satisfy legal requirements for the insurance of individual's privacy—hence, the masking of eyes of patients shown in Part I—we must question privacy on moral grounds. We believe that the so-called privacy of the back wards of these institutions contributes to suffering, for outsiders do not know the conditions in these buildings and, therefore, do little or nothing to promote improvements. When privacy contributes to suffering, we must question the ideal of privacy. When privacy contributes to suffering, it loses its significance as a cherished privilege. For those who could so reason, we do not believe that there would be many in the institutions who would object to our exposure of these frightening conditions if such exposure offered some possibility for a better life for the residents. Lastly, as we discussed this issue with a number of people we began to wonder whose privacies were being protected, those institutionalized residents or the rest of us? This leads to the second consideration.

The American people have the right to know. In spite of what we wish to know, in spite of the pain that knowing may bring to us, we have the right to be informed about any serious conditions that affect our people. There is a maturity that comes to a people when it no longer needs the protection of ignorance. Only children, with their fantasies, or sick adults, with theirs, believe that ignoring a problem can make it go away.

Our recommendations derive from many sources: our experiences prior to this study, what we observed during the study, the reactions of many astute individuals to this study, and the advice of students and colleagues. The core of our proposal was originally presented by Sarason and Gladwin a number of years ago in Sarason's book, <u>Psychological Problems in Mental Deficiency</u>, published by Harper and Row in 1959:

> It is disappointing but true that the quality of research being done in our institutions is poor. The psychological personnel are for the most part geographically, financially, and socially apart from their professional brethren. The disinterest of behavior science departments (psychology, anthropology, sociology, psychiatry) in the area of subnormal functioning makes the solution of the problem most difficult. We must frankly state that we do not have any bright ideas of how to begin to go about remedying the situation. On the assumption that this particular problem will not change markedly in the foreseeable future, it might be profitable to consider a program which would allow the institutional worker to go for extended periods to certain centers where there is an active research and training program—a center where he can possibly learn new skills and content which he could apply to research in his own setting. <u>This suggestion, however, presupposes that there will be several research centers which can offer this kind of opportunity</u>. An increment in skill and knowledge sufficient to justify this kind of effort can probably not be attained in a one- or two-week workshop, but should rather be viewed as requiring at least a half-year or year training course (p. 651).

Can one any longer ignore the needed relationship between the state institution for the mentally retarded and the state university? In addition to the emergency need for at least doubling per capita expenditures in state institutions and for reducing the sizes of institutional populations wherever and however possible, our study of this problem leads to an additional set of recommendations that may contribute to an improvement of institutional programs and facilities:

1. In each state, a board of institutional visitors should be appointed by the governor or other constituted authority. This board would be responsible for reporting directly to the highest state officials. Appointments to this board should be made regardless of political party affiliation and these appointments should be contingent on both knowledge of the broad field of human welfare and demonstrated public service. Members of this board of visitors would not be, concurrently, members of any particular institution's staff or board of trustees.

2. Within each state institution for the mentally retarded, each department (e.g., medical, psychological, educational, nursing, cottage life) should have a board of advisors. This board of advisors, through periodic visits and consultations, would know the institution and its problems intimately and, thus, be in positions to advise and assist in the resolution of difficulties. In essence, the advisory board would be organized for direct consultation and assistance to the institutional staff. As this board would not be responsible for rating institutional personnel or recommending their salary increments or promotions, it is possible that members of this board would become involved with the most pressing and severe problems of the institution—without "endangering" the positions of the staff that trusts them. In this way, it would be possible for problems currently secreted from the outside world to be given the exposure and ventilation needed for satisfactory solutions to them.

3. In each state, a state university should be given responsibility and resources to provide comprehensive in-service training and consultation for all institutional employees, from the chief administrative officer to the attendant recruit.

4. In each state, one state institution for the mentally retarded should be designated as a center for the in-service training for all personnel to be employed for state service in institutions and clinics for the mentally retarded. As a condition for employment as institutional superintendent, psychologist, teacher, nurse, or attendant the candidate would have to spend a specified period of time at the training center. His preparation program would range from a few weeks to one calendar year, depending on his background and experiences and the nature of the position he intends to assume. During this training program, the candidate would be involved in clinical experiences that relate directly to his future employment, would participate in seminars, colloquia, and other instructional experiences designed to prepare him for the sensitive and demanding activities of work with the mentally retarded. At the end of the candidate's training program, the director of this facility and his staff would rate the candidate and recommend him, or not recommend him, for employment. To the degree that this program is workable with currently employed staff, every inducement and encouragement should be provided to permit them to complete this preparation.

To some degree, all of us talk and behave as if we will not change. Yet, it is absolutely certain that we will change; what we profess now, in one way or another, we regret later. The most difficult truth each of us has to learn and live with is the knowledge that we aren't perfect. It was our intent to point out some of the more serious imperfections of institutions for the mentally retarded in this country. It is our belief that now that our indefensible practices have been laid bare for public scrutiny, men of good will from all walks of life and all professions will sit down at the planning table and seek solutions to the plight of our brethren.